EASY FITNESS FOR EASY WEIGHT LOSS - FAST

What To Actually DO To Start Losing Weight Quickly

Chris Morris

WEIGHT LOSS DOESN'T BEGIN IN THE GYM WITH A
DUMBBELL; IT STARTS IN YOUR HEAD WITH A DECISION.
—TONI SORENSEN

CONTENTS

This book is copyright protected, and it is only for personal use. You cannot amend, distribute, sell, use, quote or paraphrase any part of the content within the book without the written consent of the author or copyright owner.

Every effort has been made to make this book as complete and accurate as possible. Although the author and publisher have prepared this publication with the greatest of care, and every effort has been made to ensure its accuracy, we assume no responsibility or liability for errors, inaccuracies or omissions. You assume all risks associated with using the advice given below, with a full understanding that you, solely, are responsible for anything that may occur as a result of putting this information into action in any way, and regardless of your interpretation of the advice.

The purpose of this book is to educate. The author and publisher do not warrant that the information contained in the book is fully complete and shall not be responsible for any errors or omissions. The author and publisher shall have neither liability nor responsibility to any person or entity with respect to any loss or damage caused or alleged to be caused directly or indirectly by this book, nor do we make any claims or promises of your ability to achieve the same, or any positive, results as asserted by using any of this information.

Before you begin, please be aware that you should consult a medical professional before undertaking any form of strenuous exercise, particularly if it is unfamiliar to you. It is always a possibility that you may injure yourself while undertaking any form of physical activity. We accept no responsibility for any injuries sustained while attempting any of the exercises or activities described.

INTRODUCTION

This no-fluff book will show you how to start losing weight right now, and then maintain your new, slimmer look for good. Follow these exact steps and you <u>will</u> succeed. There's no doubt about it – as long as you <u>really</u> want to.

All of this is possible, by accomplishing increasingly easy exercises in your own home in just 15-20 minutes a day, using no specialized equipment whatsoever. Combine this with a healthy diet and secondary exercise such as walking, and your transformation will be complete.

Welcome to the **New You** program. I know just how you're feeling. Gaining weight relentlessly, seemingly without effort, and even cutting back on sugar or alcohol a little just doesn't have any effect. Have my clothes shrunk? Why am I feeling so sluggish? Why is it more effort to climb the stairs than it used to be?

So now is the time to go on a crash diet, maybe even try fasting, and lose weight that way? Wrong! *Now* is the time to build a *sustainable lifestyle choice* built around some easy exercise routines and some good old-fashioned healthy eating.

It becomes increasingly effortless after a few days, and after just one week you will feel better, you will see and feel some results, and you will want to continue. Because it is all so easy you will probably want to continue for the rest of your longer, healthier life. Why wouldn't you?

Daily exercise is what our forefathers used to do just to survive in life. Healthy eating is what they used to do simply to survive from the foods close at hand and not shipped in from a processing plant somewhere miles away.

This entire **New You** program is founded upon a sequence of easy daily exercise routines, combined with regular secondary exercise. In fact I call this part of the program 'Easy' Fitness because I originally designed it for myself and I like things easy. There's no other word for it, because that's exactly what it is.

The second part of the program involves making several small adjustments to your daily habits. It's often the case that sitting around for hours every day can be unavoidable, travelling to and from work, perhaps also for long periods during the working day, and later on surfing the net or sitting down to eat. There are changes you can make to this apparently forced inactivity, and we will go into that later on.

There is also a third element to the program, as you subtly shift towards a healthier lifestyle without needing to give up all your favourite foods. No dieting is involved as you move towards a healthy diet.

Noticeable results will start to show over the next few days and weeks, leading up to a complete transformation. Over the next 12 weeks you will quickly develop into a vastly improved version of your current self, a **New You**. In the first chapter you will soon learn how to hit the ground running, gain fitness and lose weight whenever you have a twelve-week target looming.

Summer vacation in July? No problem, pick up this book in April and you'll be confidently parading on the beach looking fit and radiant. Christmas festivities looming? Get fit for the seasonal binge by starting the program in September.

This '*Easy*' program works, every time. Stick with it and it will happen, within just 12 short weeks. The program will shape your entire future physical and mental wellbeing.

Once you have the key to fitness and health you will find that the person you have become will want to maintain a healthy lifestyle because you feel so good about yourself. Other people will compliment you, and ask you how you did it. Why would you want to regress when you know how good it feels to be at the top of your game? And the best part is that it is all so easy.

Obviously I can make no promise about your future fitness and long-term health, because I don't know you, nor do I know your current level of fitness or medical needs. What I do know, however, is that you will become fitter by closely following the advice in this book, and that becoming fit and staying fit is a fundamental aspect of living a longer and healthier life.

The exercise routines are all designed to be <u>done at home</u>, with no special equipment and <u>no visits to the gym necessary</u>. No-one need know what you are up to until you emerge from your chrysalis as a **New You**.

Each routine takes 15-20 minutes to complete. This will depend to some extent on what your current fitness level is and how quickly your body adapts as you progress through the program. Each step is carefully graduated so that you will find the exercises easier and easier as you learn them and your muscles strengthen.

It's *Easy*, but as you reach a new stage every week you will certainly be aware that you have put in some effort. Every exercise which is worth doing needs to be challenging to some degree, but you should never find yourself needing to push through the 'pain barrier'.

Your biggest challenge right now is to start. It always takes a degree of motivation to overcome a reluctance to take action, and you will be faced with this every day. As you mark your progress any motivational inertia becomes less and less, and you simply want to get on with it and feel that sense of achievement a few minutes later. After all, you have already shown some motivation in buying this book and getting this far, just on the cusp of becoming a new, fitter you. I will show you how to gain all the motivation you need to finish this program later on.

Trust me, when you have arrived at an optimized fitness level you will easily be able to take all these exercises - and more - in your stride. Once you have seen the results you will need far less motivation to keep up the momentum. Why would you not want to take just 15 or 20 minutes out of your day to maintain that newly enhanced body?

The most important advice I can give you at this introductory phase is that you owe it to yourself to complete every single one of the exercise routines set out below, on a regular basis and to the best of your ability. There is no point making excuses because then none of it will be truly worth doing. Worst of all, you will probably never get to experience the best aspect of becoming fitter - achieving that transcendent level where exercise becomes so *easy* that it is second nature. A new habit.

Once you have mastered this program, it becomes easy to step up a gear on demand. Sometimes you let it all hang out for a while, during seasonal festivities or while on vacation, but whenever you want to look good for the beach, for a brand-new job, or simply feel the need to rejuvenate yourself after a celebratory blow-out, the key to fitness will be at your fingertips. You will have the necessary foundations for fitness that I will be revealing to you over the following pages.

Let's Do This NOW...

THE FIRST STEP: DAILY EXERCISE AT HOME

There are just 16 main exercises, as well as a warming-up sequence, and the specific routines will be set out later. For now, put on some loose clothing and simply try these exercises out, one at a time. A video guide can be found here: https://easyfitnessforlife.net/free-exercise-video

If you are unfamiliar with any stretching exercises, or have rarely exerted yourself significantly for several months, even years, then go through the motions but stop short of straining to do them properly. For example, if you are unable to touch your toes, just bend forwards and reach down as far as you comfortably can.

Unless you have any physical disability, all of these exercises should be possible, and will gradually become quite easy to do in a surprisingly short time. Remember, this is an initial warm up and try out of the exercises, completing just one at a time to gauge your own fitness level at this point.

If you have any doubts about your physical health or your body's ability to accomplish these exercises please Stop Right Now and consult a physician. You should read this (page 20).

Limbering Up

Toe Touches

i)   Stand with your feet flat to the floor, approximately one foot (30cm) apart.

ii)   Gently rise onto your toes, stretching both arms upwards as far as you can reach towards the ceiling, sucking your stomach in.

iii)   Feet flat on the floor once again, bend forwards to touch your toes, or the floor if you can manage it.

iv)   Straighten up to a standing position.

Excellent exercise for the calves, bottom, upper & lower back, and arms

Lateral Body Bends

i) Stand with your feet approximately 18 inches (45 cm) apart, placing both hands behind your head.

ii) Hold your stomach in, and then bend your body sideways from the waist as far as it feels comfortable to do so. Preferably you will achieve something approaching a 45 degree angle, but you should at least feel your muscles pulling from the waist at the side, which is as it should be if you want to make a difference to your waistline.

iii) Return to the center and repeat to the opposite side.

Strengthens the spine, tones your waist and torso muscles, will help eradicate flab!

Arm Rotations

i) Raise both arms and rotate them forwards in a circular motion.

ii) Reverse the direction to complete a backwards circular motion.

Improves flexibility, tones the chest and upper back

Alternate Toe Touches

i) Stand with your feet flat to the floor, approximately one foot apart.

ii) Swing your left arm in a circular motion over your head and bend down toward the right until your hand reaches the little toe of your right foot.

iii) Straighten up, and then repeat with the right arm reaching down to your left foot.

For a trim waist, toned thighs, and a supple lower back

Running On The Spot

Jog up and down gently, lifting your legs three to four inches (7 – 10 cm) from the floor and coming down softly on your toes, for a period of 10 seconds (or count to 10 slowly).

Tones your hips and thighs, and raises your heart rate

Core Training

1. Abdominal Strength Training

i) Lie on your back, arms to the side, knees bent at 35-40 degrees, with your feet flat on the floor.

ii) Suck your stomach in, while raising your head and shoulders off the floor.

iii) Hold this position, continuing to hold your stomach in as much as possible, while also raising your legs off the floor, knees bent with the lower leg straight so that you can see your toes. Hold this position for a count of 5.

iv) Lower your legs, still bent, with a controlled motion, feeling the pull on your stomach as you do so.

v) As you lower your legs relax your head and shoulders back to the floor.

This isometric exercise is wonderful for the waistline, pulling on the lower abdominal muscles for a firm, toned stomach

2. Laid Back Kicks

i) Sit on the floor, leaning backwards with your knees bent, supporting your upper body with your hands on the floor behind you.

ii) Raise one leg 30-40 cm (12 – 16 inches) above the floor, knee still bent, and then stretch out in a kicking motion.

iii) As you do so, raise the other leg, knee bent, and kick out with this leg as you retract the first leg to a raised, knee bent, position.

Tightens the abdomen and tones the thighs

3. Thigh Squeezes

i) Stand with both legs approximately 18 inches (45 cm) apart, hands on your hips.

ii) Tighten your thigh muscles firmly, pushing your feet hard into the floor, for a count of 5. You will feel your abdomen tightening as you do so.

iii) Repeat this twice more for a total of 3 thigh squeezes.

iv) Next, widen your stance, so that your legs are approximately 24 inches (60 cm) apart, and then repeat the squeezes 3 more times, each with a count of 5.

v)   Continue to widen your legs by approximately 6 inches (15 cm) each time, squeezing 3 times on each occasion, until you are unable to maintain the position comfortably.

Tones and strengthens the thighs, and will work wonders for your walking speed

4.   Lateral Leg Raises

i)   Lie down on your right side, arms to the side, both legs together.

ii)   Raise your left leg high into the air, as high as you can, forming a V shape.

iii)   Lower your leg slowly, controlling the descent with your thigh muscles.

iv)   Lie on your right side and repeat.

Excellent exercise for the leg muscles, also your hips and waist

5.   Leg-Passing Knee Pulls

i)   Lie on your back, arms to the side, knees bent, heels on the floor.

ii)   Raise one leg, and bring it up close to your chest, clasping your hands beneath your lower thigh. Hold this position for a count of 5, then straighten your leg and raise it upwards by 90 degrees.

iii)   As you return this leg to its starting position, repeat the entire movement with your other leg, so that both legs pass in mid-air.

Excellent exercise for the thighs, bottom and hips

iv)   Reverse Curl Ups

i)   Lie on the floor, arms to the side.

ii)   Pull both knees up to your chest so that your bottom is off the floor, and cross your ankles as your knees move upwards, keeping the knees wide apart.

iii)   Firmly hold your knees or shins close to your chest with both arms, as though hugging your legs, for a count of 5, then release and straighten your legs, lowering them to the floor, uncrossed, in a controlled motion.

For a firmer bottom and thighs, also aids hip flexibility, and works your pelvic floor muscles together with your lower abdomen and lumbar area

v)   **Arm Lifts**

i)   Raise your right arm to the side, reaching high above the shoulder.

ii)   Perform the same action with your left arm.

After this gentle introduction to arm raises, it will be a great improvement to do this exercise using small weights (see page 19). I personally use two 3kg (6.6lb approx.) dumbbell-style weights, though any size ranging between 1.5kg and 3kg will do, depending on your size. This is intended for arm-toning and shoulder strength, rather than gaining massive biceps, so it is not necessary to have weights which are heavier than you can comfortably carry.

Excellent exercise for flabby or un-toned upper arms, for shoulder strength, and a good waist stretcher

vi)   **Head & Shoulder Lifts**

i)   Lie on your back, legs straight, arms to the side.

ii)   Raise your head and both shoulders off the floor, while pulling your abdominal muscles gently downwards at the same time. Hold this position for a count of 5, and then relax, slowly lowering your head and shoulders back to the floor.

A gentle exercise which tightens the abdomen and strengthens the neck

vii)   **Calf Stretches**

i)   Stand approximately 3 feet from a wall, or you could use a door frame.

ii)   Lean forward so that both arms are stretched out against the wall.

iii)   Step forward with your right foot, bending the knee, so that the toe is nearly touching the wall, keeping your left foot flat to the ground, leg straight, so that it is forming a 45% angle with the floor. Bend your right knee slightly, until you feel the calf muscle in your left leg stretching. If this feels uncomfortable then you are bending your knee too much. Hold this for a count of 5.

iv)   Now step back with the left foot, keeping it flat to the floor adjacent to your right foot, and step forward with your right leg, knee bent, so that the foot is close to the wall. Hold this for a count of 5.

Good exercise for the calf muscles, will help you power up those hills

10a. Stepped Push-ups (Male)

i)   Lie face down on the floor, legs straight, both arms bent at the elbow, palm down, in the push-up position.

ii)   Now step your right arm and your right leg out wide, and push upwards, straightening your arms as you raise your body, then control your descent to the floor.

iii)   Repeat with the left arm and leg stepped out wide.

N.B. Although this is a non-impact push-up, with less strain on your back and better shoulder movement, you may still find this exercise quite difficult at first if you have not done push-ups for a long time. If this is the case, you will find it easier to kneel than to have your legs fully extended, and continue with this version of the exercise until your arm strength has improved.

Tones the upper arms to eradicate flabbiness, as well as being excellent exercise for the shoulders and chest

10b. Diamond Push-ups (Female only). ***Before starting, read the note above.***

i)   Lie face down on the floor, arms to the side.

ii)   Move your hands together below the breastbone, forming a triangle shape with your thumb and forefingers.

iii)   Push upwards to straighten your arms at the elbow.

Tones the upper arms, counteracting arm 'jiggle', as well as being excellent exercise for the shoulders and chest

11. Roll Backs

i)   Lie on your back on the floor, arms to the side.

ii)   Raise both legs, keeping them together, and stretch them back as far as is comfortable over your head. The aim is for your toes to touch the floor behind you, but that is not possible for everyone. Try your hardest to get as close to the floor as you can. If your feet are still several inches or centimetres from the floor your effort will be equally beneficial.

iii)   As you reverse the position try to control the descent as you lower your legs to the floor, and resist the opposing force that will pull your shoulders off the floor. You should feel your lower abdomen stretching as your legs near the ground.

Good exercise to enhance the abdomen, tone thigh muscles and strengthen the lower back

12. Hand and Foot

This exercise requires more space than most, at least three feet on either side of you.

i)   Lie flat on the floor, arms by the side.

ii)   Stretch your left arm out at a right angle, palm flat to the floor.

iii)   Now swing your right leg over your body, keeping it stiff, and try to touch the tips of the fingers of your left hand with the toes of your right foot. Get as close as you can, even if your toes and fingers are not touching.

iv)   Return your right leg to your side.

v)   Now return the left arm to your side, and stretch out your right arm.

vi)   Raise your left leg and repeat (iii).

An excellent strengthening exercise for the waist muscles, good also for firming and toning your thighs

13. Pendulum Leg Swings

You will need quite a lot of space around you for this one.

i)   Lie on the floor, arms to the side.

ii)   Keeping both legs together, lift them vertically into the air, then swing to the left in a controlled motion, stopping just before your feet touch the floor.

iii)   Now swing both legs back up and over to the right.

You will immediately feel the 'pull' on your abdomen as your muscle stretches (to become better-toned over time), and this is also a great exercise for reducing any flab on your waist and hips.

14. Leg Hugs

i)   From an upright standing position step forward approximately 3 feet (nearly one metre) with your right leg.

ii)   Lean forward and clasp both hands around your bent knee, holding for 3 seconds, then straighten up and return to an upright position with both legs together.

iii)   Repeat this with your left leg.

Strengthens your thighs, toning your legs and your bottom

15. Ab Lifts

N.B. I recommend that all exercises in the *Easy Fitness* plan are best done in the morning before breakfast, but it is particularly true with this exercise, preferably with an empty stomach. Also, please note that if you currently have, or have had abdominal issues in the past, you should refer to your doctor before undertaking this powerful exercise.

i)   Stand with your feet approximately 9 - 12 inches (23 - 30 cm) apart.

ii)   Bend forwards gently and rest your hands just above each knee.

iii)   Breathe out forcefully, emptying your lungs.

iv)   Without breathing in, pull your abdomen strongly inwards, as though you are trying to pull it back to your spine, then hold this for 5-10 seconds.

v)   Breathe in gently a couple of times.

vi)   Repeat from step iii), and then do so once more, making 3 in total.

vii)   Now stand back upright again, arms loosely by the side, then raise both arms in front of you, continuing to raise them until they are high above your head, stretching up as far as you comfortably can.

viii)   Next hold your breath for about 5 seconds, feeling your abs stretch taut as you do so, then breathe in once more.

This traditional Chinese exercise is very similar to Indian yoga, and counteracts abdominal sag, as well as strengthening your diaphragm. This will aid your breathing - particularly useful for fitness exercises in general - and is also beneficial for and preventative of digestive problems

16. Full Sit Ups

N.B. If you feel significant back pain while doing this exercise you should stop immediately

i)   Lie down with your head resting on the floor, legs straight, arms across your chest with your hands resting on each shoulder.

ii)   Tighten your stomach and raise your head and shoulders off the floor as far as you can.

iii)   Keep your arms across your chest as you do so, and try as hard as you can to sit up and lean forward towards your toes.

This is a difficult – but ultimately very rewarding – exercise, and it is quite unlikely that you will be able to achieve this at your first attempt. If all you can do at this stage is to raise your head and shoulders off the floor and little more than that, then this is exactly the position I found myself in several years ago. What will happen when you persevere is that suddenly you will amaze yourself and sit right up. Maybe this week, maybe on the next week for these exercises, maybe later – but it will happen. Hard to believe at first, but when you have done this once then you can continue to do it several more times, keeping up a good rhythm. Something to show off to your friends!

When done properly, this is massively beneficial for your abdominal muscles, and will create a taut abdomen that you would never have believed possible.

Cool Down Routine

Lateral Leans
i)   Stand up straight, legs about 1 foot (30cm) apart, suck your stomach in then bend your body to the side, reaching towards the knee.
ii)   Straighten up again, and repeat the process to the other side.

Feel that pull on your waist as you stretch to each side. Another flab eliminator

Forward Bend & Stretch
N.B. This exercise will improve blood flow to the brain over time. However, you should stop immediately if you feel at all dizzy.
i)   Stand with your feet approximately 9 - 12 inches (23 - 30 cm) apart, knees slightly bent.
ii)   Lower your chin towards the collar bone, and gently roll your body forwards from the waist, arms hanging to the front, until your fingers are hanging just above your feet.
iii)   Maintaining this loose, dangling posture, chin still held in a downwards position, pull your stomach back towards the base of your spine while breathing in slowly and deeply for a count of 3, and then exhale slowly.
iv)   Now slowly unroll your body to a standing position, and imagine that your back is rolling up against a wall.

v)   When you are at your full height, chin still lowered, continue the rolling back motion to arch your back a little and raise both arms above your head.

vi)   Now repeat the earlier abdominal exercise, breathing in deeply three times for a count of 3.

vii)   Finally, relax and bring both arms down to your side in a flowing circular motion.

viii) Raise your chin and rotate your neck from side to side and up and down.

Relaxing, and terrific for your waistline, pulling on the lower abdominal muscles for a firmer stomach, while also strengthening your spine and legs

So, would you agree that these exercises are, in the main, easy to do? Bear in mind that the program involves completing just four of the core exercises in each daily routine, while steadily increasing the amount of repetitions. That's pretty much all there is to it, yet the results will be quite remarkable.

It will soon be perfectly possible to complete 15-20 of each of these four-exercise sequences within 15 minutes, while barely raising a sweat. Accomplish this and you will have simultaneously increased your body's physical capability by as much as 10 years, while at the same time feeling the pounds fall off, becoming more flexible and muscle-toned.

Now that you have started to put these words into action, it is worth considering what equipment will help you.

Equipment

One of the things I always emphasize about the **Easy Fitness** program is that no equipment is strictly necessary. There are certain items, though, which will make things even easier for you, but this is entirely for your own convenience. One thing is for sure, you definitely won't need any costly gym membership.

Here is what I use, purely by choice:

An **Exercise Mat**

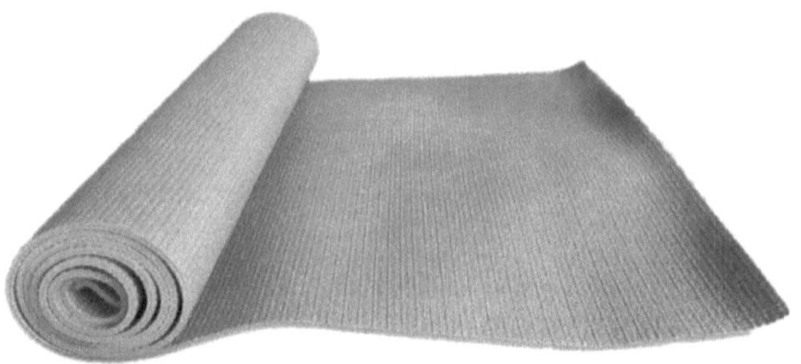

Also known as a yoga mat, such as the one shown above, this will help a lot unless you have beautifully cushioned flooring. Any discomfort you experience is best limited to pushing yourself harder to complete the exercises effectively.

A **Pedometer**

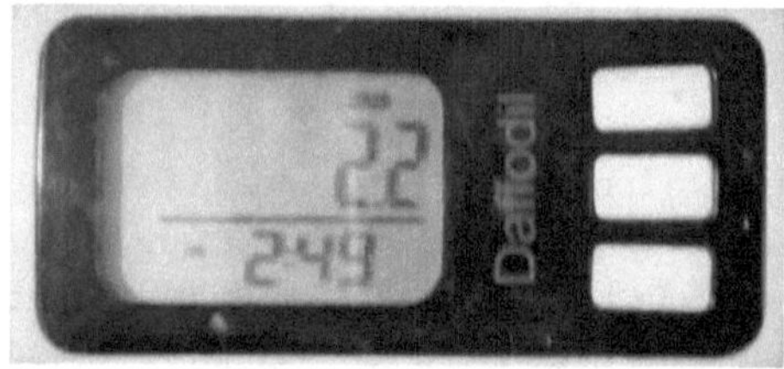

I recommend walking between 10,000 – 15,000 steps a day, depending on how much of this involves strenuous walking rather than simply shuffling around your home. Although there are many smartphone apps which will count these for you, I find that a small pedometer such as the one shown above is better. You can carry this with you wherever you go and it is amazing how the steps rack up. I regularly find myself walking 16,000 steps without any real effort, just by being active and resisting short journeys by car.

You don't actually need a pedometer if you have a regular walk that lasts 30 minutes in each direction. Add this to an active day of walking to and fro around your local environment and this should add up to at least 12,000 steps. However, having a specific target which you can reach on a pedometer or smartphone app is much more satisfying, and will also drive you on to accomplish a few more steps when you would prefer just to put your feet up. Goals are a great motivator.

An alternative to the pedometer shown above would be a Fitbit-style bracelet, which will track your movements throughout the day. You will really see the steps clock up from the moment you rise until the time you go to bed, and comparing this with a reading of the calories burned is another great motivator. The one shown here is good enough to measure steps, distance and calories, as well as waking you up 15-20 minutes earlier so that you can fit the *Easy Fitness* exercises into your busy schedule!

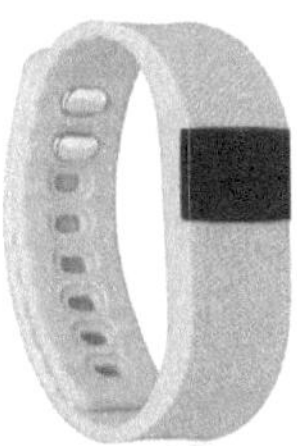

An actual Fitbit would probably be better, of course, but as with most of the 'equipment' described here, it is not strictly necessary.

Walking Shoes

It is important if you are stepping up your walking distances to 12,000 steps or more a day that you have a comfortable pair of shoes. There is no need to wear jogging or running shoes, but you should have footwear fit for the purpose when you become a frequent walker.

Dumb Bells, such as these York Barbells:

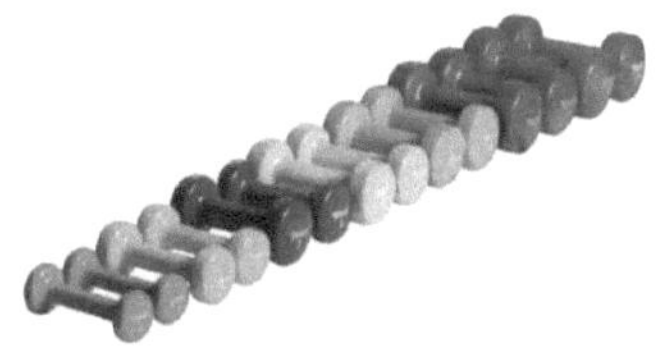

There is no weight-lifting involved in any of the exercises, but one particular exercise is great for toning the arms and flexing the chest. It is preferable to use a pair of dumb bells weighing 1.5 kg (3 pounds) or more, depending on your size, though in the past I have used saucepans and they work just as well, as long as you take care to avoid overhead light bulbs!

READ THIS BEFORE YOU START THE FULL PROGRAM

It is vital that you take account of your existing fitness level. Your brief run-through of the exercises involved was designed to inform you about your current fitness.

You should certainly consult your physician if you have not done any exercise for months. If you count yourself among those 40% of adults who fail to take as much as one brisk 10 minute walk during a month, then just by embarking on the walking aspects of this program you will be making an immediate improvement. However, be aware that starting any strenuous exercise is not recommended if you have not exercised for several months or if you know yourself to be clinically obese, <u>without having first taken medical advice.</u>

Although none of the exercise routines which follow are really difficult to complete, some of them may seem daunting at first. This will be because several – even most - may be unfamiliar to you, and to your unexercised body. For this reason they are steadily graduated from a low level according to your current fitness, and they should all be achievable by anyone who has no medical issues.

Each of them is designed to be low impact in nature, but I must stress that if you are significantly overweight, have a history of health problems, or have undertaken little or no exercise for many months, then you should definitely start off at an even lower level than recommended below. Once again, I emphasize that medical advice should first be taken if you fall into any of those categories.

Explain the workout routines to your physician, and make it clear that this program is a graduated approach to greater fitness, designed for a person of average fitness and health. No account has been taken of any pre-existing medical conditions that you and your doctor will be aware of.

In any event, I can accept no responsibility for any injuries sustained while attempting any of the exercises or activities described, and you should be aware that it will always be a possibility that you may injure yourself while undertaking any form of physical activity.

Having said all that, these disclaimers should not contradict the fact that exercise is good for you. Nevertheless, you should start at a level which suits you. Everyone is different, and the following exercises are designed for a person with a reasonable fitness level who wishes to make a positive change to their life and their future prospects. If you are able to walk at a steady pace of 2.5 - 3mph (4 - 5kph) or more for at least 20 minutes, and without any known physical impediments, then you should be able to complete the starter-level routines with ease. If you doubt that your fitness level is up to that standard, then I recommend that you start at a reduced level than set out in the course. I would suggest halving the amounts for the first two or three weeks, then aim to steadily catch up with the recommended levels within two months.

THE SECOND STEP: COMMITTING TO YOUR FUTURE

Commitment is the most important key to your success in losing weight and becoming fitter.

This is the bedrock of everything, the foundation which will keep you motivated to continue whenever you feel that doing nothing is the easier option. It shouldn't happen too often, because as I always stress, these exercises really are easy, and the diet plan is absolutely not a 'diet' which will leave you feeling hungry.

Nevertheless, we all come to a point when we feel that we just can't be bothered to make the effort. This is most likely to occur at the beginning, because the exercises may be unfamiliar, seem more difficult than they really are, and you don't feel that they are making any difference. You may also have a craving for a particular food which is not within the diet plan, even though it really is not highly restrictive.

Please don't fall into the trap of thinking that none of this is worthwhile and give up too soon. You will then be missing out on the great benefits which are just about to happen, probably within the following few days.

This is what you should do to guard against that inner voice. You should do this before you do anything else.

I know you want to lose a few pounds, be fitter, and all the things which come with that. But the real question is what, exactly, will this mean to you? Do you want to move down a clothes size or two, or perhaps fit more comfortably into the clothes you wear every day? You may even want to lose tens of pounds, and you have to start somewhere. Either way, you probably want to receive compliments on how you look.

Your motivation for wanting to improve your body is individual to you, and that means you should define in your own mind exactly what you really want to be able to gain through weight loss and greater fitness. This is your personal 'grand vision'.

Try to see in your mind's eye the body image you aspire to. It may help if you imagine the type of clothes that you feel you couldn't possibly wear right now, but would dearly love to. Perhaps you may long for a return to your more youthful body shape. You may feel that a target weight is the main aim, but try to visualize how you will look at that weight, rather than seeing it as just a number. You will know when you look and feel good, even if the scales don't necessarily reflect that.

Be as specific with your 'grand vision' as possible, write it down and refer to it daily. You could fill in the space below if you have a printed copy of this book, because you will be coming back here quite a lot over the next few weeks.

*(Complete your **grand vision** with as much detail as you can, and replace the suggestions with your own goals if you prefer.)*

I want to be..

....

I want to look like...

....

I want to weigh...

I am going to...

....

....

Challenge yourself, be aspirational, but also be realistic. Of course it's a worthwhile ambition to improve elements of your body shape, but in truth you won't be able to fundamentally alter the body you were born with. Your genes may be fixed, but whether you can fit *into* your jeans is not. That most certainly *is* under your control, as you will be learning more about later on.

The next step is vitally important. You should nominate a date to focus on for achieving your grand vision. It may be six months from now, two years from now, or even longer. Write it down, and we will start working towards that target together.

You may now be thinking that this is all just fantasy. Why should anything happen just by writing it down? The truth is, you must let go of those thoughts or they won't.

What you really should be concentrating on is the end goal, keeping it in sight all the time, so that you can measure your progress as you pass through some incremental stages, however small. You will see the snowball effect kicking in as you gain momentum, so that what once seemed a far off, daunting prospect suddenly becomes amazingly achievable, coming within reach at an increasing pace.

It is important to appreciate that although the exercises really are 'easy', and the diet plan is by no means strict, there will be times when you need to tell yourself to keep it going. The motivation to persevere when you would much prefer to give it all a miss, 'just for today', comes from keeping your end goal in sight at all times.

Initially you may feel inclined not to continue if you are not seeing instant results. This is very common. Your end goal, the grand vision, must be powerful enough to drive you on, to prevent you from taking the easy way out. The best part is that you will find 'easy fitness' and your 'easy diet plan' quickly becoming easier and easier. After just 20 or 30 days you will find that your new regime has become a habit, slotting naturally into your day.

So by now you should be forming a fixed visualization of your future self, a fixed date and a strong determination to make something happen. If you have tried and failed before, this is the time when you will succeed. The very last time you will ever have to worry about losing weight and improving your body image.

Tell Someone

Tell a friend or family member what you are planning to do. There is no need to give out all the intimate details of your grand vision, but if you tell someone about your ambition for losing weight and gaining fitness you can rely on their support and encouragement whenever your resolve may be weakening. This will add an extra boost to your resolve, a determination to demonstrate to that person that you really can do it.

THE THIRD STEP: MAKING IT ALL HAPPEN

Meet the elephant in the room. Its name is procrastination, and you have probably met him before. Right now, your personal grand vision probably seems as much a fantasy as a real elephant standing before you.

Forget the elephant for now, and think of previous New Year resolutions you have made. You probably launched into them all with the best of intentions, but then life inevitably gets in the way. One day slips by, then another a couple of days later, and after a while it all becomes pointless.

So many long-term plans end up that way. It is all too easy to delay starting, or perhaps skip a day here and there before any momentum has built. This is because the end goal on the horizon is so far away that it's almost out of sight.

After all, the end of the year seems a long way off in January, and there appears to be no rush when you have twelve months left to achieve a goal. But suddenly it's September and that once-distant deadline has become alarmingly close. With that alarm comes an enormous sense of overwhelm. A rush to the 'finishing line' leads to a panic to achieve as much as possible before it's too late. Will that result in as great an achievement as a better structured approach would have done? I don't think so.

My advice is to avoid such a haphazard scenario by deconstructing a goal into its primary elements, and then to rebuild them into a set of targets, each taking just 12 weeks. Each 12-week target leads progressively towards the end goal, which may be 6 months, 12 months or even further away.

During each 12-week phase you can reinforce to yourself the mantra that "in just 'x' weeks from now I will have achieved something really special." This will be a measurable improvement, an important step towards your grand vision.

You will find that a 12-week period channels your efforts incredibly effectively. It is just long enough to accomplish a really significant achievement, yet its duration is short enough to make the end point reassuringly close.

Each exercise plan takes full advantage of this mind-focusing yardstick which is based on some of the life-changing concepts developed in the stimulating book *The Twelve Week Year* by Brian P. Moran and Michael Lennington, which I absolutely endorse for anyone who would like to improve their life in a multitude of ways.

The fitness program and diet plan set out in the pages below target the first 12 weeks of the overarching objective which you yourself will have constructed in your own mind. In just 12 weeks' time you will be well on your way to achieving what you have set out to achieve, and it will all be so much easier.

You may have feelings of self-doubt from time to time, especially in the first few days. In fact you probably will. It's at those times when you think that you are making little or no progress that the self-reinforcing belief that you **will** do what you set out to do comes from that little voice inside. Simply revisit your objective that you defined and wrote down earlier, and believe it.

Losing weight with a good, balanced diet and *Easy Fitness* **is** easy, it really is. The only time when you may think that it is not so easy is when you first start out with some unfamiliar exercises. Your body may start to protest, but this is for the very reason that these exercises are worth doing, for the very reason that some of your muscles may have become unused to exercise. Of course, if your body is telling you that something is wrong, that is a very different thing. You should be able to recognize this difference, when you feel as though you will be causing yourself an injury if you continue.

What you should remember is that you *will* lose weight and become fit, you *will* have the improved body shape that you are setting out to achieve. You just need to allow yourself to achieve it and continue with this program until you do. I will give you all the tools you need to get there, but only you can follow through with them. Your own personal determination will self-determine your results.

Your Challenge

Your first challenge is to complete the first twelve weeks of this program. The best way to do this is to set yourself a challenging target which will stretch you, and will mark a significant step towards your end goal. For example, if your end goal is to lose 50 pounds, your twelve week target could be to lose 20 pounds.

But remember that weight in itself is not the only measurement, because it is unpredictable where the pounds will show, either on or off. You are also likely to gain muscle, which obviously weighs the same, pound for pound as a pound of fat! The good news, though, is that muscle takes up less space than fat, so you could weigh the same but the exchange of fat for muscle results in a slimmer body.

After framing your 12-week challenge you should set yourself individual mini challenges for each of the next 12 weeks, separate from the exercises themselves. The exercise routines and diet plan which I will be describing later are enough in themselves, of course, but other types of activity will broaden your fitness level and can significantly speed up your progress.

So first of all, set out your 12 Week Challenge here (or write it on the same sheet of paper as your Grand Vision):

My 12-Week Challenge is..

....

My Weekly Targets
Make each one an *action* statement
e.g.
By the end of this week –
I will have walked 30 miles
I will have cycled 50 miles
I will have eaten only fresh food this week, no junk food
I will have refrained from any alcohol for the entire 7 days
I will have swum 10 lengths of the pool every day
I will have stood up every 30 minutes during the day and moved around
By positioning these targets as accomplishments that you will have achieved, you are implying a commitment to yourself that these targets are ready and waiting to be ticked off, not merely a vague future promise to yourself.

Add as many as you like:

By the end of this week –

I will...

I will...
I will...
I will...
I will...
I will...
I will...

At the end of each week, tick off the successful accomplishment of each target. If you have missed any, score yourself out of 7 days, so that any day missed will count as 6/7. Try to make this the minimum score every week.

You will, of course, be feeling fitter as you progress through this first twelve weeks, so as the weeks go by you may wish to raise or lower your weekly targets. If you have been meeting them with ease then it's only fair to raise them a little, isn't it! It is best to wait until 4 weeks have been completed and then review the situation, and then do so again 4 weeks later. By that stage you will be amazed at how much fitter you feel, and what may have seemed challenging at first will pale into insignificance.

THE FOURTH STEP: A HEALTHY DIET

The Fast & Healthy Plan

The good news is that it is perfectly possible to lose weight and have a far healthier diet without having to deny yourself convenience foods, or having to spend more hours preparing food in the kitchen. Here is a list of quick and easy foods you can happily include in a fast, yet healthy diet:

Pasta	Rice
Bread	Strawberries and berry fruits
Unsweetened breakfast cereals	Dried fruit
Bananas	Steak
Soup in cartons or cans	Burgers
Potatoes	French fries
Eggs	Pizza
Cheese	Chinese food

There are all kinds of other foods which you probably don't consider as fast food right now, but which fit in very well with a busy lifestyle while having fantastic health benefits.

These include:

Salad	Yoghurt
Vegetables	Pulses
Fruit	

Many people like to snack or eat little and often. You may be one of them, and feel guilty about it. In actual fact, eating little and often is healthier than having just one, two, or sometimes three large meals, because our digestive systems cope better and our metabolism actually goes up when we eat like this.

So snacking is not a sin in itself. What is necessary, though, is to keep an eye on the type of snacks that you are eating. Chocolate bars and potato chips are just two examples of unhealthy snack items that can be replaced by foods that are healthier and, in fact, tastier. It's just a question of getting used to them, just like getting used to the exercise routines. Once something becomes a habit it becomes easy to maintain, and any additional treats that you may fancy from time to time cease to be a problem. You don't need to entirely give up what you enjoy for ever.

The best way of sticking to a new dietary routine is to plan ahead. Devote just 10 minutes to planning your weekly shopping and you will save an awful lot more time than simply shopping and eating on impulse.

Stock up your store cupboard with some basic items such as pasta, rice, canned pulses, tomato purée and paste, as well as spices, soy sauce and so on. Then you can quickly and easily conjure up a tasty meal in minutes when you add in some simple, fresh ingredients. Planning to buy those fresh ingredients in one visit to the shops means that you have everything organised on a week-to-week basis.

The Fast & Healthy plan is designed to fit around a busy lifestyle, so that each day of the week you choose:

One breakfast (which you can pack and eat on the move if you prefer)

One lunch - which can be eaten at home, as a packed lunch or as a takeout option

One evening meal which can be a commercial ready meal, but try to limit these to once or twice a week and ensure they total 450 calories or less

A fruit snack - each day choose one portion of any kind of fruit or, alternatively, a small glass of chilled fresh fruit juice instead.

Milk - each day you have 8 ½ oz/250 ml skimmed milk to use in tea or coffee or to drink on its own. If you do not drink milk then substitute with 4 oz/125 ml low-fat natural bio yoghurt instead to ensure you take in enough calcium. Milk for breakfast cereal is additional to this allowance.

Snacks

Each day choose 150 cal worth of snacks from the following list, mixing and matching as you like:

25 calories or less

3 dried apricots

2 fresh carrots

1 dark rye crisp bread

1 amoretti cookie

2 tablespoons of baked beans

50 calories or less

1 slice of French toast with honey

1 peach, pear or orange

1 individual light Babybel cheese

1 cheese string

1 crisp roll with peanut butter (1 teaspoon)

100 calories or less

2-cookie pack of Weight Watchers cookies

1 Shape twin pot yoghurt

1 apple and raisin cereal bar

1 Haagen-Dazs frozen yoghurt bar

1 small packet of reduced-fat potato chips

1 0.8 oz/23 g pack of Butterkist popcorn

DAILY MEALS

Choose one from each category.

Breakfasts:

- One diet fruit yoghurt, one apple, one slice of whole meal, brown or white bread, spread with a little low-fat spread and low-sugar jelly or savory spread
- One individual bio pot yoghurt, any variety, one large banana
- One medium bowl of bran flakes or cornflakes, 4 oz/125 ml skim milk, one piece of fruit
- One individual sachet or box of muesli with milk from allowance, fruit
- 6 tablespoons of baked beans on one slice of toast with a little low-fat spread
- 8 oz/225 ml low-fat natural bio yoghurt, one small sliced banana, 1 teaspoon of honey
- Half a can of whole-wheat spaghetti in tomato sauce on one slice of toast spread with a little low-fat spread

Lunches:

- One regular McDonald's hamburger (no cheese), one McDonald's pure orange juice
- Any supermarket sandwich that is 300 calories or less, fruit
- One pitta bread filled with one can of tuna in brine or spring water mixed with low fat mayonnaise or tomato sauce, chopped salad
- Any supermarket take-out salad bowl that is 300 calories or less, one slice of melon
- One can of chicken with pasta and vegetable soup, one whole-wheat roll with a little low-fat spread, fruit
- One portion take-out or supermarket pasta salad with mushrooms or vegetables, 400 calories or less
- One take-out baked potato filled with baked beans or low-fat cheese, fruit

Evening Meals

- Chicken tacos made with one chicken breast stir-fried in Old El Paso mild or hot sauce, two taco shells filled with lettuce, tomato, onion, topped with 1 tablespoon of guacamole or 1 tablespoon of Greek yoghurt.
- One shrimp or chicken chop suey (individual portion) from Chinese take-out
- One medium salmon steak, grilled or dry-fried, handful of boiled new potatoes, 4 tablespoons of peas or petit pois, 1 tablespoon hollandaise sauce or light mayonnaise
- One Weight Watchers Beef Lasagna, mixed salad
- One individual or half of a two-portion Margarita pizza
- One individual frozen cod fillet in bread crumbs, grilled, one 3.5oz/100g pack of micro fries heated in a microwave or an individual portion of fries baked in the oven, 3 tablespoons of peas or petit pois
- Two-egg omelet cooked in non-stick pan with a little oil spray and filled with 2 tablespoons of chopped ham or grated half-fat cheese, one individual pack of micro fries or individual portion of fries, salad

You have a good selection to choose from over the next 12 weeks if you stick to the Fast & Healthy Plan. However, I know how difficult it can be to isolate your meals from other members of your family, and with this in mind I can offer an entirely separate plan which you can share with other members of your family.

The Whole Family Plan

These family friendly recipes will help you attain and maintain a healthy weight, along with every other member of your family. Make sure you fill your shopping basket with plenty of healthy foods you like and that will encourage you to stick to your plan.

If you have children who are young enough not to have formed their own opinions and prejudices, this is an ideal opportunity for them to experience healthy eating too. While young children should not be on a very low-fat diet, neither should they become used to having lots of sweet foods, candy, salty and fatty snacks or sugary drinks. Young children should be given whole milk and white bread at least occasionally for its calcium content and, if they are underweight, they should be fed more energy dense foods such as carbohydrates, cheese and even French fries from time to time.

If your children take a packed lunch to school then this is an excellent opportunity to give them all those calories and nutrients they need while avoiding the calories yourself. Unless your child is overweight or obese, there's no harm in them eating plenty of sandwiches, milk, cake or muffins and even a little chocolate. Nuts and seeds are excellent for children over the age of five who do not have any allergies, and if you include a piece of fruit, you have an excellent balanced meal.

All children, including teenagers, will also benefit from a snack when they return from school or college unless they have a weight problem. If you give them a good mid-afternoon snack, especially for teens, they will then be satisfied with a less calorific meal when you all eat together later. Make sure you have a healthy snack to hand for yourself if you are preparing an earlier meal for younger children, such as fruit or crudités and a low-fat dip.

If older children and/or your partner will be eating the same meal as you in the evening, this is not a problem with this plan. You can all eat the same thing but you can simply give them bigger portions and perhaps add extra carbohydrates such as bread, potatoes, pasta, rice, etc. They can also add a little butter to their vegetables or baked potato and they can have a dessert such as fruit and cream or yoghurt.

Never tell your family that you're on a slimming diet, but rather that you're going to begin to eat more healthily. Most healthy adults and children hate the idea of slimming and the low-calorie foods that usually entails and to be honest they have a good point. But with this diet, there is absolutely no need to consider yourself to be dieting or slimming. In fact you are simply boosting your health and, in the process, making yourself feel and look better.

Make sure that you plan ahead as this is absolutely vital to the success of this plan. If you spend a little time each week planning your menus, you will save a great deal more time when shopping or in the kitchen.

Always be aware of what you're eating and why. There will come a point when you find that you can easily resist eating to excess or even at all unless you are genuinely hungry and therefore need the food. Remember that weight gain is rarely caused just by what you eat at your main meals, but rather by what you eat in between and when away from home - in other words, snacks.

Of course there will always be special occasions when you want to produce a more elaborate meal. That's absolutely fine and you can regularly include that within your regime, knowing that it will not throw you off course.

If budget is a consideration, keep in mind that healthy food is not actually more expensive. Buy in-season salads, fruit and vegetables as well as meat and fish, and you will find that you are not spending more than you usually do. If you also include a good amount of carbohydrates such as bread, potatoes, pasta and rice, you will not only have staples that the entire family will be happy to eat but you will also find that these are extremely good value.

There are a few more expensive items within this plan but there is absolutely no need to choose them if you don't want to or if they don't fit within your budget. Remember that if you're cutting down on fattening foods such as cookies, cakes, candy and desserts, you will have more money to spare for the extra fruit and vegetables that you will be buying.

Unlimited Foods

The following foods are unlimited on this plan:

Drinks: water, mineral water, herbal teas, green tea, tea and coffee with milk from your daily allowance (no sugar), lemon juice, zero calorie soft drinks.

Foods: carrots, cucumbers, salad and leafy greens, leafy green vegetables.

Herbs, sauces and spices: fresh or dried herbs and spices, lemon juice, tomato purée or paste, low-fat stock (cubes or powder), vinegar, light soy sauce, oil-free French dressing and other low calorie salad dressings.

Daily milk allowance: you have a daily milk allowance of 8 ½ fluid oz/250 ml skim milk for use in tea or coffee or on its own as a drink. If you do not take milk then replace this with one 4 oz/125 ml pot of natural low-fat yoghurt. Milk for breakfast cereals is in addition to this allowance.

Fruit: one portion of fruit in this plan means one medium piece of fruit, a small banana, or two small fruits such as plums or satsumas; alternatively, you could try a medium bowl of small berry fruits such as strawberries, or a small handful of grapes, or a medium bowl of fresh fruit salad.

Bread: one slice of bread in this plan means one slice from a large, medium cut loaf with a little low-fat spread. This can be toasted if preferred.

DAILY MEALS

Choose one from each meal category.

Breakfasts:
- One slice of bread, 2 teaspoons of low-sugar jelly or jam, one large banana, one small glass of fresh fruit juice
- One English muffin spread with low-fat spread and 2 teaspoons of low-sugar jelly or jam, one portion of fruit
- One twin pot of bio yoghurt, one slice of toast with 2 teaspoons of low-sugar jelly or jam, one small fruit
- One medium boiled or poached egg, one slice of bread, one glass of fresh fruit juice
- One medium bowl of low-fat natural bio yoghurt, a handful of muesli, one portion of fruit, one spoonful of sesame seeds

- Small bowl of cornflakes or bran flakes with 4 oz/125 ml low-fat natural yoghurt, one chopped apple and 1 teaspoon of sesame seeds, one glass of fresh fruit juice
- One medium bowl of porridge made with water, skim milk to cover, 1 teaspoon of honey, slice of toast

Lunches:

- Any take-out sandwich, 300 calories or less, one portion of fruit
- One small cooked chicken breast with one large mixed salad and 4 tablespoons of cooked rice or pasta, mixed with oil-free French dressing and chopped dried apricots, one fruit fromage frais
- One carton of fresh soup, one small whole-wheat roll or one slice bread
- One McDonald's hamburger (no cheese), one McDonald's pure fruit juice
- One small low-fat, stone baked vegetable pizza, green salad
- One take-out pasta or rice salad, 300 calories or less, one glass of fresh fruit juice
- Sandwich made with two slices of bread filled with 3.5 oz/100 g tuna in brine or water, drained, one tablespoon of low-fat mayonnaise, salad, one portion of fruit

Evening meals:

- Four cod fillet fish fingers, grilled or baked, 3 tablespoons of mashed potato, 4 tablespoons of peas, one portion of fruit
- Two-egg omelette cooked in a non-stick pan sprayed with oil, filled with mushrooms or grilled red peppers, 3.5 oz/100 g oven fries, peas or salad
- One small lean steak, 2 tablespoons of new potatoes, 4 tablespoons of sweetcorn or green beans, one portion of fruit
- 4.5 oz/125 g portion roast lamb or pork, two roast potatoes, one spoonful of mint or apple sauce, unlimited leafy green vegetables, 2 tablespoons of thin gravy

- One medium chicken breast (skin removed), grilled or baked, 3 tablespoons of new potatoes, 4 tablespoons of sweetcorn or peas, one large banana
- One medium baked potato filled with one small can of baked beans, top with 2 tablespoons of grated half fat hard cheese, salad
- Two large, low-fat sausages, grilled, 3 tablespoons of mashed potato, unlimited leafy green vegetables or 4 tablespoons of baked beans, one portion of fruit

Snacks and treats:
- One medium glass of wine or ½ pint/275 ml bottle cider or beer
- Two dark rye crisp breads spread with one tablespoon of peanut butter
- One small bag of reduced-fat potato chips
- One pack of 2 chocolate chip Weight Watchers cookies
- One apple and raisin chewy bar

Simply sticking solidly to either of the above Plans for just 30 days should reduce your weight by 10 pounds. Continue for the full length of your 12-week Exercise Plan and, in addition to the energy expended through the exercises, you could be 30 pounds lighter, allowing for my earlier comments regarding muscle.

Bear in mind, however, that it is best not to be obsessed with scales. There is always a time lag before the full effects are revealed, and your weight is not so important as how you look, and how you feel. You will know when you feel healthy, and your friends and family will be sure to tell you when you are looking good. That is the true measure of your success with the *Easy Fitness* plan.

The link between Exercise, Diet and Health
When you have reached your desired weight you can incorporate elements of these diet plans into a broader, well-balanced diet. Maintain the recommended average calorie level for your age and sex, while continuing to follow the exercises laid out in this program, and you will then be placing yourself firmly on the path towards a long and healthy life.

THE FIFTH STEP: EXERCISE STARTS HERE

You should by now have assessed your own fitness level, based on the ease with which you took on and accomplished the trial exercises in Chapter One – The First Step.

For those of you who found them far too easy, you probably count among the fittest readers of this book, and are really looking for a fast way of regaining a little lost fitness and losing some weight as quickly as possible. You should start at Level Three, one step down from my *Extreme* Exercise Program.

If the initial round of exercises was a little challenging but you managed them without making a huge effort, then you should start at Level Two. This is for people who may be in their thirties or forties, perhaps younger, who have let their fitness slide for several weeks or months and have noticed the effect this has had on their overweight body. You could also try them as a fairly fit fifty-something who sees room for improvement – but be prepared to lower your sights towards Level One.

Level One is for people who are very unfit, who have done little or no exercise apart from casual walks of less than a mile, probably for many months or even years. Also anyone over fifty or sixty who feels the need to start off slowly and progress to Level Two when ready.

Each of these levels are fundamentally based on similar exercises, and you should see similar effects within 12 weeks, amounting to a noticeable improvement in your fitness level, weight, and a general awareness that your body has reacted positively to your new regime. This will be matched by an improved sense of well-being and an enhanced outlook on life.

Enough of the reading. A New You starts here:

LEVEL ONE

Start at Level One if you have done no significant exercise for several months or more, other than walking an average of one mile or less a day. Also, anyone over the age of 50 should start at Level One unless you consider yourself to be fitter than average.

If the exercise routine feels too easy after the first couple of days then experiment with moving up to Level Two.

LEVEL TWO

Begin with Level Two if you consider yourself to be reasonably fit but have lapsed and let it all hang out for a month or more. Also, anyone over the age of 40 should start with Level Two and assess how much effort is involved.

If the exercise routine feels too easy after the first couple of days then experiment with moving up to Level Three. You may well find it quite challenging!

LEVEL THREE

Level Three should only be attempted by anyone who is under the age of forty and has been quite fit for long periods but has recently put on weight and/or let their fitness lapse for a month or two.

The routines can be challenging, particularly at first, but there is no reason why a reasonably fit person should not be able to achieve them. Age is not necessarily a barrier, and I can accomplish them with ease at the age of 63, but it may be dangerous for anyone unused to exercise.

Whichever level you begin at, you should ultimately be able to complete the Level Three exercise routines after progressing through this book.

*

Remind yourself of your main Vision, remind yourself of your separate Weekly Targets, and get ready to launch into:

WEEK ONE

DAY ONE

This is the day when you take control of your future fitness. Try as hard as you can, but don't push yourself excessively at this stage. Be prepared for a longer session than will be usual, while you familiarize yourself with the exercises.

(Refer back to the full Exercise Descriptions in Chapter One – The First Step, and you can also download a video guide to the exercises here: *https://easyfitnessforlife.net/free-exercise-video*).

Limbering Up

Toe Touches
(Level 1 – L1) Begin with 5 in total
(Level 2 – L2) Begin with 10 in total
(Level 3 – L3) Begin with 15 in total

Arm Rotations
(L1) Raise both arms and rotate them forwards in a circular motion, 5 times. Repeat with 5 times backwards.
(L2) 5 forwards, 5 backwards
(L3) 8 forwards, 8 backwards

Lateral Body Bends
Bend your body sideways from the waist as far as it feels comfortable to do so.
(L1) Begin with 5 bends to each side
(L2) 10 each side
(L3) 15 each side

Alternate Toe Touches
(L1) Start with five toe touches to each side
(L2) 5 to each side
(L3) 8 to each side

Running On The Spot

(L1) Raise your heartbeat a little for a period of 30 seconds (or count to 30 slowly).
(L2) 30 seconds
(L3) 45 seconds

Core Training

Abdominal Strength Training
(L1) Start off with 3 in total
(L2) 5 in total
(L3) 10 in total

Laid Back Kicks
(L1) An alternate kicking motion, 10 times with each leg
(L2) 15 with each leg
(L3) 20 with each leg

Thigh Squeezes
Widen your legs by approximately 6 inches (15 cm) each time, squeezing your thighs 3 times on each occasion, until you are unable to maintain the position comfortably.
(L1) Repeat 4 more times for a total of 5
(L2) 6 sets of thigh squeezes
(L3) 8 sets of thigh squeezes

Lateral Leg Raises
(L1) Lie down on your right side, raise your left leg high into the air, forming a V shape. Repeat 9 more times, then turn onto your left side and repeat the process.
(L2) 15 with each leg
(L3) 20 with each leg

Cooling Down

Lateral Leans
(L1) Bend your body to the side, reaching towards the knee, straighten up and repeat the process to the other side, for a total of 5 leans each side.
(L2) 10 to each side
(L3) 15 to each side

Forward Bend & Stretch

(L1) Begin with 3 bends, but Stop Immediately if you feel at all dizzy.
(L2) Begin with 3 bends.
(L3) Begin with 5 bends.

This completes your exercise routine for the day, and will probably have taken longer than 20 minutes. Don't despair – you <u>will</u> speed up!

Now walk up and down for approximately 30 seconds as your pulse rate reduces.

Additional Exercise: Just by walking on a regular basis, as specified below (Daily Steps), you can reduce your rate of physical decline by as much as 50%, which is quite an amazing figure. Making a point of walking, using the stairs rather than escalator, and avoiding being seated for long periods (over 1 hour) will all help improve your general fitness. Alternatively you could also Cycle or Swim regularly.

Daily Steps: 10,000 minimum (approximately 5 miles, depending on your stride length).

DAY TWO
Don't be surprised if your body is feeling a little stiff after the unfamiliar exercises yesterday. This is perfectly normal, and unless you are feeling any undue pain, proceed gently with your second day. Any stiffness will disappear soon after beginning, and it will become easier over time. Starting is difficult, continuing is easy.

Limbering Up
Running On The Spot - (L1) 30 seconds (L2) 30 seconds (L3) 50 seconds
Toe Touches - (L1) 5 (L2) 10 (L3) 16
Arm Rotations - (L1) 5 forwards, 5 backwards (L2) 5/5 (L3) 9/9
Lateral Body Bends - (L1) 5 to each side (L2) 10/10 (L3) 16/16
Alternate Toe Touches - (L1) 5 to each side (L2) 5/5 (L3) 9/9

Core Training

Abdominal Strength Training - (L1) 3 (L2) 5 (L3) 11
Laid Back Kicks - (L1) 10 with each leg (L2) 15 (L3) 22
Thigh Squeezes - (L1) 5 sets (L2) 6 sets (L3) 9 sets
Lateral Leg Raises - (L1) 10 on each side (L2) 15 (L3) 22

Cool Down

Lateral Leans - (L1) 5 each side (L2) 10 each side (L3) 16 each side
Forward Bend & Stretch - (L1) 3 (L2) 3 (L3) 5

Walk up and down for approximately 30 seconds as your pulse rate reduces.
Daily Steps: 10,000 minimum (approximately 5 miles)

DAY THREE

Limbering Up

Running On The Spot - (L1) 35 seconds (L2) 35 seconds (L3) 55 seconds
Toe Touches - (L1) 6 (L2) 11 (L3) 17
Arm Rotations - (L1) 6 forwards, 6 backwards (L2) 6/6 (L3) 10/10
Lateral Body Bends - (L1) 6 to each side (L2) 11/11 (L3) 17/17
Alternate Toe Touches - (L1) 6 to each side (L2) 6/6 (L3) 10/10

Core Training

Leg-Passing Knee Pulls
(L1) A new exercise today. Repeat these alternating knee pulls to complete 3 sequences with each leg.
(L2) 5
(L3) 10

Abdominal Strength Training - (L1) 4 (L2) 6 (L3) 12
Thigh Squeezes - (L1) 6 sets (L2) 7 sets (L3) 10 sets

Ab Lifts
Another new exercise today, and as I mentioned earlier, this particular exercise is best done in the morning, with an empty stomach. Also, please note that if you currently have, or have had abdominal issues in the past, you should refer to your doctor before undertaking this powerful exercise.

(L1) Complete a sequence of 3 Ab Lifts.
(L2) 4 Ab Lifts
(L3) 5 Ab Lifts

Cooling Down

Lateral Leans - (L1) 6 each side (L2) 11 each side (L3) 17 each side
Forward Bend & Stretch - (L1) 3 (L2) 3 (L3) 5

Walk up and down for approximately 30 seconds as your pulse rate reduces.
Daily Steps: 10,000 minimum (approximately 5 miles)

DAY FOUR
A REST DAY – Limber Up Only

Running On The Spot - (L1) 35 seconds (L2) 35 seconds (L3) 60 seconds
Toe Touches - (L1) 6 (L2) 11 (L3) 18
Arm Rotations - (L1) 6 forwards, 6 backwards (L2) 6/6 (L3) 11/11
Lateral Body Bends - (L1) 6 to each side (L2) 11/11 (L3) 18/18
Alternate Toe Touches - (L1) 6 to each side (L2) 6/6 (L3) 11/11

DAY FIVE
Limbering Up

Running On The Spot - (L1) 40 seconds (L2) 40 seconds (L3) 70 seconds
Toe Touches - (L1) 7 (L2) 12 (L3) 19
Arm Rotations - (L1) 7 forwards, 7 backwards (L2) 7/7 (L3) 12/12
Lateral Body Bends - (L1) 7 to each side (L2) 12/12 (L3) 19/19
Alternate Toe Touches - (L1) 7 to each side (L2) 7/7 (L3) 12/12

Core Training

Leg-Passing Knee Pulls - (L1) 3 (L2) 5 (L3) 11
Abdominal Strength Training - (L1) 4 (L2) 6 (L3) 13
Thigh Squeezes - (L1) 6 sets (L2) 7 (L3) 10 sets
Ab Lifts - (L1) 3 (L2) 4 (L3) 6

Cooling Down

Lateral Leans - (L1) 6 each side (L2) 11 (L3) 18 each side
Forward Bend & Stretch - (L1) 3 (L2) 3 (L3) 6

Walk up and down for approximately 30 seconds as your pulse rate reduces.

Daily Steps: 10,000 minimum (approximately 5 miles)

DAY SIX

Limbering Up

Running On The Spot – (L1) 40 seconds (L2) 40 secs (L3) 80 seconds
Toe Touches – (L1) 7 (L2) 12 (L3) 20
Arm Rotations – (L1) 7 forwards, 7 backwards (L2) 7/7 (L3) 13/13
Lateral Body Bends – (L1) 7 to each side (L2) 12/12 (L3) 20/20
Alternate Toe Touches – (L1) 7 to each side (L2) 7/7 (L3) 13/13

Core Training

Abdominal Strength Training – (L1) 5 (L2) 7 (L3) 14
Laid Back Kicks – (L1) 11 with each leg (L2) 16 (L3) 24
Thigh Squeezes – (L1) 7 sets (L2) 8 (L3) 10 sets
Lateral Leg Raises – (L1) 11 on each side (L2) 16 (L3) 24

Cool Down

Lateral Leans – (L1) 7 each side (L2) 12 (L3) 19 each side
Forward Bend & Stretch – (L1) 3 (L2) 3 (L3) 6

Walk up and down for approximately 30 seconds as your pulse rate reduces.
Daily Steps: 10,000 minimum (approximately 5 miles)

DAY SEVEN

Limbering Up

Running On The Spot – (L1) 45 seconds (L2) 45 secs (L3) 90 seconds
Toe Touches – (L1) 8 (L2) 13 (L3) 22
Arm Rotations – (L1) 8 forwards, 8 backwards (L2) 8/8 (L3) 14/14
Lateral Body Bends – (L1) 8 to each side (L2) 13/13 (L3) 20/20
Alternate Toe Touches – (L1) 8 to each side (L2) 8/8 (L3) 14/14

Core Training

Leg-Passing Knee Pulls – (L1) 4 (L2) 6 (L3) 12

Abdominal Strength Training – (L1) 5 (L2) 7 (L3) 15
Thigh Squeezes – (L1) 7 sets (L2) 8 (L3) 10 sets
Ab Lifts – (L1) 4 (L2) 5 (L3) 7

Cooling Down

Lateral Leans – (L1) 7 each side (L2) 12 (L3) 20 each side
Forward Bend & Stretch – (L1) 3 (L2) 3 (L3) 6

Walk up and down for approximately 30 seconds as your pulse rate reduces.
Daily Steps: 10,000 minimum (approximately 5 miles)

Tough going so far, or as easy as it says at the top of this book? If you have completed **all** the exercises to the best of your ability, and also hit an 85% strike rate on your own Weekly Targets then you will start to notice some early signs of real improvement over the next week. You will be loosening up well and, even though it is early days, you may just feel some of your clothes hanging differently on you.

WEEK TWO

DAY ONE

Limbering Up

Running On The Spot – (L1) 45 seconds (L2) 45 seconds (L3) 100 seconds
Toe Touches – (L1) 8 (L2) 13 (L3) 24
Arm Rotations – (L1) 8 forwards, 8 backwards (L2) 8/8 (L3) 15/15
Lateral Body Bends – (L1) 8 to each side (L2) 13/13 (L3) 20/20
Alternate Toe Touches – (L1) 8 to each side (L2) 8/8 (L3) 15/15

Core Training

Reverse Curl Ups
(L1) Start with 3 Curl Ups (L2) 5 (L3) 8

Laid Back Kicks – (L1) 11 with each leg (L2) 16 (L3) 26

Arm Lifts (preferably with weights of between 1.5kg – 3kg)

(L1) Begin with 3 to each side, then 4 lifts with both arms simultaneously, totalling 10 rounds in all.
(L2) 5/5/5 (15 in all)
(L3) 6/6/8 (20 in all)

Head & Shoulder Lifts
(L1) Begin with 5 of these exercises (L2) 10 (L3) 15

Cooling Down

Lateral Leans – (L1) 8 each side (L2) 13 each side (L3) 20 each side
Forward Bend & Stretch – (L1) 4 (L2) 4 (L3) 7

Walk up and down for approximately 30 seconds as your pulse rate reduces.
Daily Steps: 10,000 minimum (approximately 5 miles)

DAY TWO
Rest Day

Limbering Up Only

Running On The Spot – (L1) 50 seconds (L2) 50 secs (L3) 110 seconds
Toe Touches – (L1) 9 (L2) 14 (L3) 26
Arm Rotations – (L1) 9 forwards, 9 backwards (L2) 9/9 (L3) 16/16
Lateral Body Bends – (L1) 9 to each side (L2) 14 each side (L3) 20/20
Alternate Toe Touches – (L1) 9 to each side (L2) 9/9 (L3) 16/16

Daily Steps: 10,000 minimum (approximately 5 miles)

DAY THREE

Limbering Up

Running On The Spot – 50 seconds (L2) 50 seconds (L3) 120 seconds
Toe Touches – (L1) 9 (L2) 14 (L3) 28
Arm Rotations – (L1) 9 forwards, 9 backwards (L2) 9/9 (L3) 17/17
Lateral Body Bends – (L1) 9 to each side (L2) 14/14 (L3) 20/20
Alternate Toe Touches – (L1) 9 to each side (L2) 9/9 (L3) 17/17

Core Training

Reverse Curl Ups – (L1) 3 (L2) 5 (L3) 9
Laid Back Kicks – (L1) 12 with each leg (L2) 17 each leg (L3) 28
Arm Lifts – (L1) 10 (3 Left 3 Right 4 together) (L2) 15 (5/5/5) (L3) 22 (7/7/8)
Head & Shoulder Lifts – (L1) 5 (L2) 10 (L3) 16

Cool Down

Lateral Leans – (L1) 8 each side (L2) 13 each side (L3) 20 each side
Forward Bend & Stretch – (L1) 4 (L2) 4 (L3) 7

Walk up and down for approximately 30 seconds as your pulse rate reduces.
Daily Steps: 10,000 minimum (approximately 5 miles)

DAY FOUR

Limbering Up

Running On The Spot – (L1) 55 seconds (L2) 55 seconds (L3) 120 seconds
Toe Touches – (L1) 10 (L2) 15 (L3) 30
Arm Rotations – (L1) 10 forwards, 10 backwards (L2) 10/10 (L3) 18/18
Lateral Body Bends – (L1) 10 to each side (L2) 15/15 (L3) 20/20
Alternate Toe Touches – (L1) 10 to each side (L2) 10/10 (L3) 18/18

Core Training

Leg-Passing Knee Pulls – (L1) 4 (L2) 6 (L3) 13
Calf Stretches
(L1) Repeat this exercise to complete 5 with each leg
(L2) 7 with each leg
(L3) 10 with each leg

Lateral Leg Raises – (L1) 11 on each side (L2) 16 each side (L3) 26 each side
Stepped Push-ups (Male)
(L1) Start off with two sets, one with left arm and leg stepped out, then the right
arm and leg, and repeat
(L2) 5 sets
(L3) 10 sets

Diamond Push-ups (Female only)
(L1) Begin with 3 push-ups (L2) 5 push-ups (L3) 8 push-ups

Cooling Down

Lateral Leans - (L1) 9 each side (L2) 14 each side (L3) 20 each side
Forward Bend & Stretch - (L1) 4 (L2) 4 (L3) 7

Walk up and down for approximately 30 seconds as your pulse rate reduces.
Daily Steps: 10,000 minimum (approximately 5 miles)

DAY FIVE

Limbering Up

Running On The Spot - (L1) 55 seconds (L2) 55 seconds (L3) 120 seconds
Toe Touches - (L1) 10 (L2) 15 (L3) 30
Arm Rotations - (L1) 10 forwards, 10 backwards (L2) 10/10 (L3) 19/19
Lateral Body Bends - (L1) 10 to each side (L2) 15 each side (L3) 20/20
Alternate Toe Touches - (L1) 10 to each side (L2) 10/10 (L3) 19/19

Core Training

Leg-Passing Knee Pulls - (L1) 5 (L2) 7 (L3) 14
Calf Stretches - (L1) 5 (L2) 7 (L3) 11 each leg
Lateral Leg Raises - (L1) 12 on each side (L2) 17 each side (L3) 28 each side
Stepped Push Ups (male) - (L1) 3 (L2) 5 (L3) 11 sets
Diamond Push Ups (female) - (L1) 3 (L2) 5 (L3) 9

Cooling Down

Lateral Leans - (L1) 9 each side (L2) 14 each side (L3) 20 each side
Forward Bend & Stretch - (L1) 4 (L2) 4 (L3) 7

Walk up and down for approximately 30 seconds as your pulse rate reduces.
Daily Steps: 10,000 minimum (approximately 5 miles)

DAY SIX

Limbering Up

Running On The Spot – (L1) 60 seconds (L2) 60 seconds (L3) 120 seconds
Toe Touches – (L1) 11 (L2) 16 (L3) 30
Arm Rotations – (L1) 11 forwards, 11 backwards (L2) 11/11 (L3) 20/20
Lateral Body Bends – (L1) 11 to each side (L2) 16/16 (L3) 20/20
Alternate Toe Touches – (L1) 10 to each side (L2) 10/10 (L3) 20/20

Core Training

Reverse Curl Ups – (L1) 4 (L2) 6 (L3) 10
Laid Back Kicks – (L1) 12 with each leg (L2) 17 each leg (L3) 30
Arm Lifts – (L1) 11 (3 Left, 3 Right, 5 together) (L2) 16 (5/5/6) (L3) 24 (8/8/8)
Head & Shoulder Lifts – (L1) 6 (L2) 11 (L3) 17

Cooling Down

Lateral Leans – (L1) 10 each side (L2) 15 each side (L3) 20 each side
Forward Bend & Stretch – (L1) 4 (L2) 4 (L3) 7

Walk up and down for approximately 30 seconds as your pulse rate reduces.
Daily Steps: 10,000 minimum (approximately 5 miles)

DAY SEVEN

Limbering Up

Running On The Spot – (L1) 60 seconds (L2) 60 seconds (L3) 120 seconds
Toe Touches – (L1) 11 (L2) 16 (L3) 30
Arm Rotations – (L1) 11 forwards, 11 backwards (L2) 11/11 (L3) 20/20
Lateral Body Bends – (L1) 11 to each side (L2) 16 each side (L3) 20/20
Alternate Toe Touches – (L1) 10 to each side (L2) 10/10 (L3) 20/20

Core Training

Leg-Passing Knee Pulls – (L1) 5 (L2) 7 (L3) 15
Calf Stretches – (L1) 6 (L2) 8 (L3) 12 each leg
Lateral Leg Raises – (L1) 12 on each side (L2) 17 each side (L3) 30
Stepped Push Ups (male) – (L1) 4 (L2) 6 (L3) 12 sets
Diamond Push Ups (female) – (L1) 4 (L2) 6 (L3) 10

Cooling Down

Lateral Leans – (L1) 10 each side (L2) 15 each side (L3) 20 each side
Forward Bend & Stretch – (L1) 4 (L2) 4 (L3) 7

Walk up and down for approximately 30 seconds as your pulse rate reduces.
Daily Steps: 10,000 minimum (approximately 5 miles)

Now we are really making progress...

WEEK THREE

DAY ONE

Limbering Up

Running On The Spot – (L1) 65 seconds (L2) 65 seconds (L3) 120 seconds
Toe Touches – (L1) 12 (L2) 17 (L3) 30
Arm Rotations – (L1) 12 forwards, 12 backwards (L2) 12/12 (L3) 20/20
Lateral Body Bends – (L1) 12 to each side (L2) 17 each side (L3) 20/20
Alternate Toe Touches – (L1) 10 to each side (L2) 10 each side (L3) 20/20

Core Training

Abdominal Strength Training – (L1) 6 (L2) 8 (L3) 16
Roll Backs
(L1) Begin with 3 Roll Backs (L2) 5 (L3) 6
Arm Lifts – (L1) 11 (3/3/5) (L2) 16 (5/5/6) (L3) 26 (8/8/10)
Thigh Squeezes – (L1) 8 sets (L2) 9 sets (L3) 10 sets

Cooling Down

Lateral Leans – (L1) 11 each side (L2) 16 each side (L3) 20 each side
Forward Bend & Stretch – (L1) 5 (L2) 5 (L3) 7

Walk up and down for approximately 30 seconds as your pulse rate reduces.
Daily Steps: 10,000 minimum (approximately 5 miles)

DAY TWO

Rest Day: Limbering Up Only

Running On The Spot – (L1) 65 seconds (L2) 65 seconds (L3) 120 seconds
Toe Touches – (L1) 12 (L2) 17 (L3) 30
Arm Rotations – (L1) 12 forwards, 12 backwards (L2) 12/12 (L3) 20/20
Lateral Body Bends – (L1) 12 to each side (L2) 17 each side (L3) 20/20
Alternate Toe Touches – (L1) 10 to each side (L2) 10/10 (L3) 20/20

Daily Steps: 10,000 minimum (approximately 5 miles)

DAY THREE

Limbering Up

Running On The Spot – (L1) 70 seconds (L2) 70 seconds (L3) 120 seconds
Toe Touches – (L1) 13 (L2) 18 (L3) 30
Arm Rotations – (L1) 13 forwards, 13 backwards (L2) 13/13 (L3) 20/20
Lateral Body Bends – (L1) 13 to each side (L2) 18/18 (L3) 20/20
Alternate Toe Touches – (L1) 10 to each side (L2) 10/10 (L3) 20/20

Core Training

Abdominal Strength Training – (L1) 6 (L2) 8 (L3) 17
Roll Backs – (L1) 3 (L2) 5 (L3) 7
Arm Lifts – (L1) 12 (4 Left, 4 Right, 4 together) (L2) 17 (5/5/7) (L3) 28 (9/9/10)
Thigh Squeezes – (L1) 8 sets (L2) 9 sets (L3) 10 sets

Cooling Down

Lateral Leans – (L1) 11 each side (L2) 16 each side (L3) 20 each side
Forward Bend & Stretch – (L1) 5 (L2) 5 (L3) 7

Walk up and down for approximately 30 seconds as your pulse rate reduces.
Daily Steps: 10,000 minimum (approximately 5 miles)

DAY FOUR

Limbering Up

Running On The Spot – (L1) 70 seconds (L2) 70 seconds (L3) 120 seconds
Toe Touches – (L1) 13 (L2) (L2) 18 (L3) 30
Arm Rotations – (L1) 13 forwards, 13 backwards (L2) 13/13 (L3) 20/20
Lateral Body Bends – (L1) 13 to each side (L2) 18/18 (L3) 20/20
Alternate Toe Touches – (L1) 10 to each side (L2) 10/10 (L3) 20/20

Core Training

Calf Stretches – (L1) 6 (L2) 8 (L3) 13 each leg
Hand to Foot
(L1) Start with 5 exercises to each side (L2) 10 each side (L3) 12 each side
Laid Back Kicks – (L1) 13 with each leg (L2) 18 (L3) 32
Ab Lifts – (L1) 4 (L2) 5 (L3) 8

Cooling Down

Lateral Leans – (L1) 12 each side (L2) 17 each side (L3) 20 each side
Forward Bend & Stretch – (L1) 5 (L2) 5 (L3) 7

Walk up and down for approximately 30 seconds as your pulse rate reduces.
Daily Steps: 10,000 minimum (approximately 5 miles)

DAY FIVE

Limbering Up

Running On The Spot – (L1) 75 seconds (L2) 75 seconds (L3) 120 seconds
Toe Touches – (L1) 14 (L2) 19 (L3) 30
Arm Rotations – (L1) 14 forwards, 14 backwards (L2) 14/14 (L3) 20/20
Lateral Body Bends – (L1) 14 to each side (L2) 19/19 (L3) 20/20
Alternate Toe Touches – (L1) 10 to each side (L2) 10/10 (L3) 20/20

Core Training

Calf Stretches – (L1) 7 (L2) 9 (L3) 14 each leg
Hand to Foot – (L1) 5 (L2) 10 (L3) 13
Laid Back Kicks – (L1) 13 with each leg (L2) 18 each leg (L3) 34
Ab Lifts – (L1) 5 (L2) 6 (L3) 8

Cooling Down

Lateral Leans – (L1) 12 each side (L2) 17 each side (L3) 20 each side
Forward Bend & Stretch – (L1) 5 (L2) 5 (L3) 7

Walk up and down for approximately 30 seconds as your pulse rate reduces.
Daily Steps: 10,000 minimum (approximately 5 miles)

DAY SIX

Limbering Up

Running On The Spot – (L1) 75 seconds (L2) 75 seconds (L3) 120 seconds
Toe Touches – (L1) 14 (L2) 19 (L3) 30
Arm Rotations – (L1) 14 forwards, 14 backwards (L2) 14/14 (L3) 20/20
Lateral Body Bends – (L1) 14 to each side (L2) 19 each side (L3) 20/20
Alternate Toe Touches – (L1) 10 to each side (L2) 10/10 (L3) 20/20

Core Training

Abdominal Strength Training – (L1) 7 (L2) 9 (L3) 18
Roll Backs – (L1) 4 (L2) 6 (L3) 8
Arm Lifts – (L1) 12 (4 Left, 4 Right, 4 together) (L2) 17 (5/5/7) (L3) 30 (10/10/10)
Thigh Squeezes – (L1) 9 sets (L2) 10 sets (L3) 10 sets

Cooling Down

Lateral Leans – (L1) 13 each side (L2) 18 each side (L3) 20 each side
Forward Bend & Stretch – (L1) 5 (L2) 5 (L3) 7

Walk up and down for approximately 30 seconds as your pulse rate reduces.
Daily Steps: 10,000 minimum (approximately 5 miles)

DAY SEVEN

Limbering Up

Running On The Spot – (L1) 80 seconds (L2) 80 seconds (L3) 120 seconds
Toe Touches – (L1) 15 (L2) 20 (L3) 30
Arm Rotations – (L1) 15 forwards, 15 backwards (L2) 15/15 (L3) 20/20

Lateral Body Bends - (L1) 15 to each side (L2) 20/20 (L3) 20/20
Alternate Toe Touches - (L1) 10 to each side (L2) 10/10 (L3) 20/20

Core Training

Calf Stretches - (L1) 7 (L2) 9 (L3) 15 each leg
Hand to Foot - (L1) 6 (L2) 11 (L3) 14
Laid Back Kicks - (L1) 14 with each leg (L2) 19 (L3) 36
Ab Lifts - (L1) 5 (L2) 6 (L3) 8

Cooling Down

Lateral Leans - (L1) 13 each side (L2) 18 each side (L3) 20 each side
Forward Bend & Stretch - (L1) 5 (L2) 5 (L3) 7

Walk up and down for approximately 30 seconds as your pulse rate reduces.
Daily Steps: 10,000 minimum (approximately 5 miles)

WEEK FOUR

DAY ONE

Limbering Up

Running On The Spot - (L1) 80 seconds (L2) 80 seconds (L3) 120 seconds
Toe Touches - (L1) 15 (L2) 20 (L3) 30
Arm Rotations - (L1) 15 forwards, 15 backwards (L2) 15/15 (L3) 20/20
Lateral Body Bends - (L1) 15 to each side (L2) 20/20 (L3) 20/20
Alternate Toe Touches - (L1) 10 to each side (L2) 10/10 (L3) 20/20

Core Training

Reverse Curl Ups - (L1) 4 (L2) 6 (L3) 11
Arm Lifts - (L1) 13 (4 Left, 4 Right, 5 together) (L2) 18 (6/6/6) (L3) 32 (10/10/12)
Head & Shoulder Lifts - (L1) 6 (L2) 11 (L3) 18

Full Sit Ups
This is one of the most difficult exercises at first for most people. As mentioned previously, if you feel significant back pain while doing this exercise you should stop immediately.

(L1) Begin with 3 Sit Ups, and in the likely event that you are unable to manage a complete sit up at the first attempt, do the best you can, even if all you can do at this stage is to raise your head and shoulders off the floor and little more than that. It does get easier!
(L2) 5
(L3) 10

Cooling Down

Lateral Leans - (L1) 14 each side (L2) 19 each side (L3) 20 each side
Forward Bend & Stretch - (L1) 5 (L2) 5 (L3) 7

Walk up and down for approximately 30 seconds as your pulse rate reduces.
Daily Steps: 10,000 minimum (approximately 5 miles)

DAY TWO

Limbering Up

Running On The Spot - (L1) 85 seconds (L2) 85 seconds (L3) 120 seconds
Toe Touches - (L1) 16 (L2) 21 (L3) 30
Arm Rotations - (L1) 16 forwards, 16 backwards (L2) 16/16 (L3) 20/20
Lateral Body Bends - (L1) 16 to each side (L2) 20/20 (L3) 20/20
Alternate Toe Touches - (L1) 10 to each side (L2) 10/10 (L3) 20/20

Core Training

Reverse Curl Ups - (L1) 5 (L2) 7 (L3) 12
Arm Lifts - (L1) 13 (4 Left, 4 Right, 5 together) (L2) 18 (6/6/6) (L3) 34 (11/11/12)
Head & Shoulder Lifts - (L1) 7 (L2) 12 (L3) 20
Full Sit Ups - (L1) 3 (L2) 5 (L3) 11

Cooling Down

Lateral Leans - (L1) 14 each side (L2) 19 each side (L3) 20 each side
Forward Bend & Stretch - (L1) 5 (L2) 5 (L3) 7

Walk up and down for approximately 30 seconds as your pulse rate reduces.
Daily Steps: 10,000 minimum (approximately 5 miles)

DAY THREE

Limbering Up Only

Running On The Spot – (L1) 85 seconds (L2) 85 seconds (L3) 120 seconds
Toe Touches – (L1) 16 (L2) 21 (L3) 30
Arm Rotations – (L1) 16 forwards, 16 backwards (L2) 16/16 (L3) 20/20
Lateral Body Bends – (L1) 16 to each side (L2) 20/20 (L3) 20/20
Alternate Toe Touches – (L1) 10 to each side (L2) 10/10 (L3) 20/20

Daily Steps: 10,000 minimum (approximately 5 miles)

DAY FOUR

Limbering Up

Running On The Spot – (L1) 90 seconds (L2) 90 seconds (L3) 120 seconds
Toe Touches – (L1) 17 (L2) 22 (L3) 30
Arm Rotations – (L1) 17 forwards, 17 backwards (L2) 17/17 (L3) 20/20
Lateral Body Bends – (L1) 17 to each side (L2) 20/20 (L3) 20/20
Alternate Toe Touches – (L1) 10 to each side (L2) 10/10 (L3) 20/20

Core Training

Abdominal Strength Training – (L1) 7 (L2) 9 (L3) 19
Lateral Leg Raises – (L1) 13 on each side (L2) 18 each side (L3) 32 each side
Calf Stretches – (L1) 8 (L2) 10 (L3) 15 each leg
Pendulum Leg Swings
(L1) You will need quite a lot of space around you, swinging your legs from one side to the other, completing 3 to each side
(L2) 5 each side
(L3) 8 each side

Cooling Down

Lateral Leans - (L1) 15 each side (L2) 20 each side (L3) 20 each side
Forward Bend & Stretch - (L1) 5 (L2) 5 (L3) 7

Walk up and down for approximately 30 seconds as your pulse rate reduces.
Daily Steps: 10,000 minimum (approximately 5 miles)

DAY FIVE

Limbering Up

Running On The Spot - (L1) 90 seconds (L2) 90 seconds (L3) 120 seconds
Toe Touches - (L1) 17 (L2) 22 (L3) 30
Arm Rotations - (L1) 17 forwards, 17 backwards (L2) 17/17 (L3) 20/20
Lateral Body Bends - (L1) 17 to each side (L2) 20/20 (L3) 20/20
Alternate Toe Touches - (L1) 10 to each side (L2) 10/10 (L3) 20/20

Core Training

Abdominal Strength Training - (L1) 8 (L2) 10 (L3) 20
Lateral Leg Raises - (L1) 13 on each side (L2) 18 each side (L3) 34
Calf Stretches - (L1) 8 (L2) 10 (L3) 15
Pendulum Leg Swings - (L1) 3 (L2) 5 (L3) 9

Cooling Down

Lateral Leans - (L1) 15 each side (L2) 20 each side (L3) 20 each side
Forward Bend & Stretch - (L1) 5 (L2) 5 (L3) 7

Walk up and down for approximately 30 seconds as your pulse rate reduces.
Daily Steps: 10,000 minimum (approximately 5 miles)

DAY SIX

Limbering Up

Running On The Spot - (L1) 95 seconds (L2) 95 seconds (L3) 120 seconds
Toe Touches - (L1) 18 (L2) 23 (L3) 30
Arm Rotations - (L1) 18 forwards, 18 backwards (L2) 18/18 (L3) 20/20
Lateral Body Bends - (L1) 18 to each side (L2) 20/20 (L3) 20/20
Alternate Toe Touches - (L1) 10 to each side (L2) 10/10 (L3) 20/20

Core Training

Reverse Curl Ups – (L1) 5 (L2) 7 (L3) 13
Arm Lifts – (L1) 14 (4 Left, 4 Right, 6 together) (L2) 19 (6/6/7) (L3) 36 (12/12/12)
Head & Shoulder Lifts – (L1) 7 (L2) 12 (L3) 22
Full Sit Ups – (L1) 4 (L2) 6 (L3) 12

Cool Down

Lateral Leans – (L1) 16 each side (L2) 20 each side (L3) 20 each side
Forward Bend & Stretch – (L1) 5 (L2) 5 (L3) 7

Walk up and down for approximately 30 seconds as your pulse rate reduces.
Daily Steps: 10,000 minimum (approximately 5 miles)

DAY SEVEN

Limbering Up

Running On The Spot – (L1) 95 seconds (L2) 95 seconds (L3) 120 seconds
Toe Touches – (L1) 18 (L2) 23 (L3) 30
Arm Rotations – (L1) 18 forwards, 18 backwards (L2) 18/18 (L3) 20/20
Lateral Body Bends – (L1) 18 to each side (L2) 20/20 (L3) 20/20
Alternate Toe Touches – (L1) 10 to each side (L2) 10/10 (L3) 20/20

Core Training

Abdominal Strength Training – (L1) 8 (L2) 10 (L3) 20
Lateral Leg Raises – (L1) 14 on each side (L2) 19 (L3) 36 each side
Calf Stretches – (L1) 9 (L2) 11 (L3) 15
Pendulum Leg Swings – (L1) 4 (L2) 6 (L3) 10

Cool Down

Lateral Leans – (L1) 16 each side (L2) 20 each side (L3) 20 each side
Forward Bend & Stretch – (L1) 5 (L2) 5 (L3) 7

Walk up and down for approximately 30 seconds as your pulse rate reduces.
Daily Steps: 10,000 minimum (approximately 5 miles)

Four Weeks completed. Congratulations on showing the determination to get this far. Now it is time to take stock and review your Weekly Targets which you set just over 4 weeks ago. Are you achieving an 85% strike rate (about 6 days out of 7, for example), or has it been a struggle? Now is the time to re-align yourself with your main vision, your overriding goal, and re-set your targets to make sure you get there. If you have to set your targets a little lower then that is OK. It is difficult to set a target at exactly the right level until you get used to setting them. The same applies if you have found your targets not challenging enough (achieving 100% every week without any real effort, for example). Try again, and make it better this time. We are nearly ready to go again, into the fifth week and beyond!

How about the main Exercise Plan? You should be achieving at least an 85% strike rate, and preferably 100% if you are to gain the full benefits from this program. If you are achieving 100% completion then that is ideal, and it will become easier and easier for you to take on the exercises, even as they are increasing in number.

WEEK FIVE

DAY ONE

Limbering Up

Running On The Spot - (L1) 100 seconds (L2) 100 seconds (L3) 120 seconds
Toe Touches - (L1) 19 (L2) 24 (L3) 30
Arm Rotations - (L1) 19 forwards, 19 backwards (L2) 19/19 (L3) 20/20
Lateral Body Bends - (L1) 19 to each side (L2) 20/20 (L3) 20/20
Alternate Toe Touches - (L1) 10 to each side (L2) 10/10 (L3) 20/20

Core Training

Leg-Passing Knee Pulls - (L1) 6 (L2) 8 (L3) 15
Ab Lifts - (L1) 6 (L2) 7 (L3) 8

Stepped Push Ups (male) - (L1) 4 (L2) 6 (L3) 13 sets
Diamond Push Ups (female) - (L1) 4 (L2) 6 (L3) 11
Thigh Squeezes - (L1) 9 sets (L2)10 sets (L3) 10 sets

Cooling Down

Lateral Leans - (L1) 17 each side (L2) 20 each side (L3) 20 each side
Forward Bend & Stretch - (L1) 5 (L2) 5 (L3) 7

Walk up and down for approximately 30 seconds as your pulse rate reduces.
Daily Steps: 10,000 minimum (approximately 5 miles)

DAY TWO

Limbering Up

Running On The Spot - (L1) 100 seconds (L2) 100 seconds (L3) 120 seconds
Toe Touches - (L1) 19 (L2) 24 (L3) 30
Arm Rotations - (L1) 19 forwards, 19 backwards (L2) 19/19 (L3) 20/20
Lateral Body Bends - (L1) 19 to each side (L2) 20/20 (L3) 20/20
Alternate Toe Touches - (L1) 10 to each side (L2) 10/10 (L3) 20/20

Core Training

Leg-Passing Knee Pulls - (L1) 6 (L2) 8 (L3) 15
Ab Lifts - (L1) 6 (L2) 7 (L3) 8
Stepped Push Ups (male) - (L1) 5 (L2) 7 (L3) 14 sets
Diamond Push Ups (female) - (L1) 5 (L2) 7 (L3) 12
Thigh Squeezes - (L1) 10 sets (L2) 10 sets (L3) 10 sets

Cooling Down

Lateral Leans - (L1) 17 each side (L2) 20 each side (L3) 20 each side
Forward Bend & Stretch - (L1) 5 (L2) 5 (L3) 7

Walk up and down for approximately 30 seconds as your pulse rate reduces.
Daily Steps: 10,000 minimum (approximately 5 miles)

DAY THREE

Limbering Up

Running On The Spot - (L1) 105 seconds (L2) 105 seconds (L3) 120 seconds
Toe Touches - (L1) 20 (L2) 25 (L3) 30
Arm Rotations - (L1) 20 forwards, 20 backwards (L2) 20/20 (L3) 20/20
Lateral Body Bends - (L1) 20 to each side (L2) 20/20 (L3) 20/20
Alternate Toe Touches - (L1) 10 to each side (L2) 10/10 (L3) 20/20

Core Training

Laid Back Kicks - (L1) 14 with each leg (L2) 19 each leg (L3) 38
Roll Backs - (L1) 4 (L2) 6 (L3) 9
Arm Lifts - (L1) 14 (4 Left, 4 Right, 6 together) (L2) 19 (6/6/7) (L3) 36 (12/12/12)
Full Sit Ups - (L1) 4 (L2) 6 (L3) 13

Cooling Down

Lateral Leans - (L1) 18 each side (L2) 20 each side (L3) 20 each side
Forward Bend & Stretch - (L1) 5 (L2) 5 (L3) 7

Walk up and down for approximately 30 seconds as your pulse rate reduces.
Daily Steps: 10,000 minimum (approximately 5 miles)

DAY FOUR

Limbering Up Only

Running On The Spot - (L1) 105 seconds (L2) 105 seconds (L3) 120 seconds
Toe Touches - (L1) 20 (L2) 25 (L3) 30
Arm Rotations - (L1) 20 forwards, 20 backwards (L2) 20/20 (L3) 20/20
Lateral Body Bends - (L1) 20 to each side (L2) 20/20 (L3) 20/20
Alternate Toe Touches - (L1) 10 to each side (L2) 10/10 (L3) 20/20

Daily Steps: 10,000 minimum (approximately 5 miles)

DAY FIVE

Limbering Up

Running On The Spot - (L1) 110 seconds (L2) 110 seconds (L3) 120 seconds

Toe Touches – (L1) 20 (L2) 26 (L3) 30
Arm Rotations – (L1) 20 forwards, 20 backwards (L2) 20/20 (L3) 20/20
Lateral Body Bends – (L1) 20 to each side (L2) 20/20 (L3) 20/20
Alternate Toe Touches – (L1) 10 to each side (L2) 10/10 (L3) 20/20

Core Training

Laid Back Kicks – (L1) 15 with each leg (L2) 20 each leg (L3) 40
Roll Backs – (L1) 5 (L2) 7 (L3) 9
Arm Lifts – (L1) 15 (5 Left, 5 Right, 5 together) (L2) 20 (6/6/8) (L3) 36 (12/12/12)
Full Sit Ups – (L1) 5 (L2) 7 (L3) 14

Cooling Down

Lateral Leans – (L1) 18 each side (L2) 20 each side (L3) 20 each side
Forward Bend & Stretch – (L1) 5 (L2) 5 (L3) 7

Walk up and down for approximately 30 seconds as your pulse rate reduces.
Daily Steps: 10,000 minimum (approximately 5 miles)

DAY SIX

Limbering Up

Running On The Spot – (L1) 110 seconds (L2) 110 seconds (L3) 120 seconds
Toe Touches – (L1) 20 (L2) 26 (L3) 30
Arm Rotations – (L1) 20 forwards, 20 backwards (L2) 20/20 (L3) 20/20
Lateral Body Bends – (L1) 20 to each side (L2) 20/20 (L3) 20/20
Alternate Toe Touches – (L1) 10 to each side (L2) 10/10 (L3) 20/20

Core Training

Leg-Passing Knee Pulls – (L1) 7 (L2) 9 (L3) 15
Ab Lifts – (L1) 7 (L2) 8 (L3) 8
Stepped Push Ups (male) – (L1) 5 (L2) 7 (L3) 15 sets
Diamond Push Ups (female) – (L1) 5 (L2) 7 (L3) 13
Thigh Squeezes – (L1) 10 sets (L2) 10 sets (L3) 10 sets

Cooling Down

Lateral Leans - (L1) 19 each side (L2) 20 each side (L3) 20 each side
Forward Bend & Stretch - (L1) 5 (L2) 5 (L3) 7

Walk up and down for approximately 30 seconds as your pulse rate reduces.
Daily Steps: 10,000 minimum (approximately 5 miles)

DAY SEVEN

Limbering Up

Running On The Spot - (L1) 115 seconds (L2) 115 seconds (L3) 120 seconds
Toe Touches - (L1) 20 (L2) 27 (L3) 30
Arm Rotations - (L1) 20 forwards, 20 backwards (L2) 20/20 (L3) 20/20
Lateral Body Bends - (L1) 20 to each side (L2) 20/20 (L3) 20/20
Alternate Toe Touches - (L1) 10 to each side (L2) 10/10 (L3) 20/20

Core Training

Laid Back Kicks - (L1) 15 with each leg (L2) 20 (L3) 40
Roll Backs - (L1) 5 (L2) 7 (L3) 9
Arm Lifts - (L1) 15 (5 Left, 5 Right, 5 together) (L2)20 (6/6/8) (L3) 36 (12/12/12)
Full Sit Ups - (L1) 5 (L2) 7 (L3) 15

Cooling Down

Lateral Leans - (L1) 19 each side (L2) 20 each side (L3) 20 each side
Forward Bend & Stretch - (L1) 5 (L2) 5 (L3) 7

Walk up and down for approximately 30 seconds as your pulse rate reduces.
Daily Steps: 10,000 minimum (approximately 5 miles)

WEEK SIX

DAY ONE

Limbering Up

Running On The Spot - (L1) 115 seconds (L2) 115 seconds (L3) 120 seconds

Toe Touches – (L1) 20 (L2) 27 (L3) 30
Arm Rotations – (L1) 20 forwards, 20 backwards (L2) 20/20 (L3) 20/20
Lateral Body Bends – (L1) 20 to each side (L2) 20/20 (L3) 20/20
Alternate Toe Touches – (L1) 10 to each side (L2) 10/10 (L3) 20/20

Core Training

Reverse Curl Ups – (L1) 6 (L2) 8 (L3) 14
Hand to Foot – (L1) 6 (L2) 11 (L3) 15
Head & Shoulder Lifts – (L1) 8 (L2) 13 (L3) 24
Ab Lifts – (L1) 7 (L2) 8 (L3) 8

Cool Down

Lateral Leans – (L1) 20 each side (L2) 20 each side (L3) 20 each side
Forward Bend & Stretch – (L1) 5 (L2) 5 (L3) 7

Walk up and down for approximately 30 seconds as your pulse rate reduces.
Daily Steps: 10,000 minimum (approximately 5 miles)

DAY TWO

Limbering Up

Running On The Spot – (L1) 120 seconds (L2) 120 seconds (L3) 120 seconds
Toe Touches – (L1) 20 (L2) 28 (L3) 30
Arm Rotations – (L1) 20 forwards, 20 backwards (L2) 20/20 (L3) 20/20
Lateral Body Bends – (L1) 20 to each side (L2) 20/20 (L3) 20/20
Alternate Toe Touches – (L1) 10 to each side (L2) 10/10 (L3) 20/20

Core Training

Reverse Curl Ups – (L1) 6 (L2) 8 (L3) 15
Hand to Foot – (L1) 7 (L2) 12 (L3) 16
Head & Shoulder Lifts – (L1) 8 (L2) 13 (L3) 25
Ab Lifts – (L1) 7 (L2) 8 (L3) 8

Cooling Down

Lateral Leans – (L1) 20 each side (L2) 20 each side (L3) 20 each side

Forward Bend & Stretch – (L1) 5 (L2) 5 (L3) 7

Walk up and down for approximately 30 seconds as your pulse rate reduces.
Daily Steps: 10,000 minimum (approximately 5 miles)

DAY THREE
Limbering Up

Running On The Spot – (L1) 120 seconds (L2) 120 seconds (L3) 120 seconds
Toe Touches – (L1) 20 (L2) 28 (L3) 30
Arm Rotations – (L1) 20 forwards, 20 backwards (L2) 20/20 (L3) 20/20
Lateral Body Bends – (L1) 20 to each side (L2) 20/20 (L3) 20/20
Alternate Toe Touches – (L1) 10 to each side (L2) 10/10 (L3) 20/20

Core Training

Stepped Push Ups (male) – (L1) 6 (L2) 8 (L3) 17 sets
Diamond Push Ups (female) – (L1) 6 (L2) 8 (L3) 14
Lateral Leg Raises – (L1) 14 on each side (L2) 19 each side (L3) 38 each side
Calf Stretches – (L1) 9 (L2) 11 (L3) 15
Leg Hugs
The final new exercise! Complete the sequence for a total of three for each leg.
(L1) 3
(L2) 3
(L3) 10
Cooling Down

Lateral Leans – (L1) 20 each side (L2) 20 each side (L3) 20 each side
Forward Bend & Stretch – (L1) 5 (L2) 5 (L3) 7

Walk up and down for approximately 30 seconds as your pulse rate reduces.
Daily Steps: 10,000 minimum (approximately 5 miles)

DAY FOUR
Limbering Up Only

Running On The Spot – (L1) 120 seconds (L2) 120 seconds (L3) 120 seconds
Toe Touches – (L1) 20 (L2) 28 (L3) 30

Arm Rotations - (L1) 20 forwards, 20 backwards (L2) 20/20 (L3) 20/20
Lateral Body Bends - (L1) 20 to each side (L2) 20/20 (L3) 20/20
Alternate Toe Touches - (L1) 10 to each side (L2) 10/10 (L3) 20/20

Daily Steps: 10,000 minimum (approximately 5 miles)

DAY FIVE

Limbering Up

Running On The Spot - (L1) 120 seconds (L2) 120 seconds (L3) 120 seconds
Toe Touches - (L1) 20 (L2) 28 (L3) 30
Arm Rotations - (L1) 20 forwards, 20 backwards (L2) 20/20 (L3) 20/20
Lateral Body Bends - (L1) 20 to each side (L2) 20/20 (L3) 20/20
Alternate Toe Touches - (L1) 10 to each side (L2) 10/10 (L3) 20/20

Core Training

Stepped Push Ups (male) - (L1) 6 (L2) 8 (L3) 19 sets
Diamond Push Ups (female) - (L1) 6 (L2) 8 (L3) 15
Lateral Leg Raises - (L1) 15 on each side (L2) 20 each side (L3) 40 each side
Calf Stretches - (L1) 10 (L2) 12 (L3) 15
Leg Hugs - (L1) 3 (L2) 5 (L3) 11

Cooling Down

Lateral Leans - (L1) 20 each side (L2) 20 each side (L3) 20 each side
Forward Bend & Stretch - (L1) 5 (L2) 5 (L3) 7

Walk up and down for approximately 30 seconds as your pulse rate reduces.
Daily Steps: 10,000 minimum (approximately 5 miles)

DAY SIX

Limbering Up

Running On The Spot - (L1) 120 seconds (L2) 120 seconds (L3) 120 seconds
Toe Touches - (L1) 20 (L2) 28 (L3) 30

Arm Rotations - (L1) 20 forwards, 20 backwards (L2) 20/20 (L3) 20/20
Lateral Body Bends - (L1) 20 to each side (L2) 20/20 (L3) 20/20
Alternate Toe Touches - (L1) 10 to each side (L2) 10/10 (L3) 20/20

Core Training

Reverse Curl Ups - (L1) 7 (L2) 9 (L3) 15
Hand to Foot - (L1) 7 (L2) 12 (L3) 18
Head & Shoulder Lifts - (L1) 9 (L2) 14 (L3) 25
Ab Lifts - (L1) 7 (L2) 8 (L3) 8

Cooling Down

Lateral Leans - (L1) 20 each side (L2) 20 each side (L3) 20 each side
Forward Bend & Stretch - (L1) 5 (L2) 5 (L3) 7

Walk up and down for approximately 30 seconds as your pulse rate reduces.
Daily Steps: 10,000 minimum (approximately 5 miles)

DAY SEVEN

Limbering Up

Running On The Spot - (L1) 120 seconds (L2) 120 seconds (L3) 120 seconds
Toe Touches - (L1) 20 (L2) 28 (L3) 30
Arm Rotations - (L1) 20 forwards, 20 backwards (L2) 20/20 (L3) 20/20
Lateral Body Bends - (L1) 20 to each side (L2) 20/20 (L3) 20/20
Alternate Toe Touches - (L1) 10 to each side (L2) 10/10 (L3) 20/20

Core Training

Stepped Push Ups (male) - (L1) 7 (L2) 9 (L3) 21 sets
Diamond Push Ups (female) - (L1) 7 (L2) 9 (L3) 15
Lateral Leg Raises - (L1) 15 (L2) 20 (L3) 40 each side
Calf Stretches - (L1) 10 (L2) 12 (L3) 15
Leg Hugs - (L1) 4 (L2) 6 (L3) 12

Cooling Down

Lateral Leans - (L1) 20 each side (L2) 20 each side (L3) 20 each side

Forward Bend & Stretch – (L1) 5 (L2) 5 (L3) 7

Walk up and down for approximately 30 seconds as your pulse rate reduces.
Daily Steps: 10,000 minimum (approximately 5 miles)

WEEK SEVEN

DAY ONE

Limbering Up

Running On The Spot – (L1) 120 seconds (L2) 120 seconds (L3) 120 seconds
Toe Touches – (L1) 20 (L2) 28 (L3) 30
Arm Rotations – (L1) 20 forwards, 20 backwards (L2) 20/20 (L3) 20/20
Lateral Body Bends – (L1) 20 to each side (L2) 20/20 (L3) 20/20
Alternate Toe Touches – (L1) 10 to each side (L2) 10/10 (L3) 20/20

Core Training

Hand to Foot – (L1) 8 (L2) 13 (L3) 20
Abdominal Strength Training – (L1) 9 (L2) 11 (L3) 20
Leg-Passing Knee Pulls – (L1) 7 (L2) 9 (L3) 15
Pendulum Leg Swings – (L1) 4 (L2) 6 (L3) 12

Cooling Down

Lateral Leans – (L1) 20 each side (L2) 20 each side (L3) 20 each side
Forward Bend & Stretch – (L1) 5 (L2) 5 (L3) 7

Walk up and down for approximately 30 seconds as your pulse rate reduces.
Daily Steps: 10,000 minimum (approximately 5 miles)

DAY TWO

Limbering Up

Running On The Spot – (L1) 120 seconds (L2) 120 seconds (L3) 120 seconds
Toe Touches – (L1) 20 (L2) 28 (L3) 30

Arm Rotations - (L1) 20 forwards, 20 backwards (L2) 20/20 (L3) 20/20
Lateral Body Bends - (L1) 20 to each side (L2) 20/20 (L3) 20/20
Alternate Toe Touches - (L1) 10 to each side (L2) 10/10 (L3) 20/20

Core Training

Hand to Foot - (L1) 8 (L2) 13 (L3) 20
Abdominal Strength Training - (L1) 9 (L2) 11 (L3) 20
Leg-Passing Knee Pulls - (L1) 8 (L2) 10 (L3) 15
Pendulum Leg Swings - (L1) 5 (L2) 7 (L3) 14

Cooling Down

Lateral Leans - (L1) 20 each side (L2) 20 each side (L3) 20 each side
Forward Bend & Stretch - (L1) 5 (L2) 5 (L3) 7

Walk up and down for approximately 30 seconds as your pulse rate reduces.
Daily Steps: 10,000 minimum (approximately 5 miles)

DAY THREE
Limbering Up

Running On The Spot - (L1) 120 seconds (L2) 120 seconds (L3) 120 seconds
Toe Touches - (L1) 20 (L2) 28 (L3) 30
Arm Rotations - (L1) 20 forwards, 20 backwards (L2) 20/20 (L3) 20/20
Lateral Body Bends - (L1) 20 to each side (L2) 20/20 (L3) 20/20
Alternate Toe Touches - (L1) 10 to each side (L2) 10/10 (L3) 20/20

Core Training

Roll Backs - (L1) 6 (L2) 8 (L3) 9
Calf Stretches - (L1) 10 (L2) 13 (L3) 15
Thigh Squeezes - (L1) 10 sets (L2) 10 sets (L3) 10 sets
Full Sit Ups - (L1) 6 (L2) 8 (L3) 16

Cooling Down

Lateral Leans - (L1) 20 each side (L2) 20 each side (L3) 20 each side
Forward Bend & Stretch - (L1) 5 (L2) 5 (L3) 7

Walk up and down for approximately 30 seconds as your pulse rate reduces.
Daily Steps: 10,000 minimum (approximately 5 miles)

DAY FOUR

Limbering Up Only

Running On The Spot – (L1) 120 seconds (L2) 120 seconds (L3) 120 seconds
Toe Touches – (L1) 20 (L2) 28 (L3) 30
Arm Rotations – (L1) 20 forwards, 20 backwards (L2) 20/20 (L3) 20/20
Lateral Body Bends – (L1) 20 to each side (L2) 20/20 (L3) 20/20
Alternate Toe Touches – (L1) 10 to each side (L2) 10/10 (L3) 20/20

Daily Steps: 10,000 minimum (approximately 5 miles)

DAY FIVE

Limbering Up

Running On The Spot – (L1) 120 seconds (L2) 120 seconds (L3) 120 seconds
Toe Touches – (L1) 20 (L2) 30 (L3) 30
Arm Rotations – (L1) 20 forwards, 20 backwards (L2) 20/20 (L3) 20/20
Lateral Body Bends – (L1) 20 to each side (L2) 20/20 (L3) 20/20
Alternate Toe Touches – (L1) 10 to each side (L2) 10/10 (L3) 20/20

Core Training

Roll Backs – (L1) 6 (L2) 8 (L3) 9
Calf Stretches – (L1) 10 (L2) 13 (L3) 15
Thigh Squeezes – (L1) 10 sets (L2) 10 sets (L3) 10 sets
Full Sit Ups – (L1) 6 (L2) 8 (L3) 17

Cooling Down

Lateral Leans – (L1) 20 each side (L2) 20 each side (L3) 20 each side
Forward Bend & Stretch – (L1) 5 (L2) 5 (L3) 7

Walk up and down for approximately 30 seconds as your pulse rate reduces.
Daily Steps: 10,000 minimum (approximately 5 miles)

DAY SIX

Limbering Up

Running On The Spot - (L1) 120 seconds (L2) 120 seconds (L3) 120 seconds
Toe Touches - (L1) 20 (L2) 30 (L3) 30
Arm Rotations - (L1) 20 forwards, 20 backwards (L2) 20/20 (L3) 20/20
Lateral Body Bends - (L1) 20 to each side (L2) 20/20 (L3) 20/20
Alternate Toe Touches - (L1) 10 to each side (L2) 10/10 (L3) 20/20

Core Training

Hand to Foot - (L1) 9 (L2) 14 (L3) 20
Abdominal Strength Training - (L1) 10 (L2) 12 (L3) 20
Leg-Passing Knee Pulls - (L1) 8 (L2) 10 (L3) 15
Pendulum Leg Swings - (L1) 5 (L2) 7 (L3) 16

Cooling Down

Lateral Leans - (L1) 20 each side (L2) 20 each side (L3) 20 each side
Forward Bend & Stretch - (L1) 5 (L2) 5 (L3) 7

Walk up and down for approximately 30 seconds as your pulse rate reduces.
Daily Steps: 10,000 minimum (approximately 5 miles)

DAY SEVEN

Limbering Up

Running On The Spot - (L1) 120 seconds (L2) 120 seconds (L3) 120 seconds
Toe Touches - (L1) 20 (L2) 30 (L3) 30
Arm Rotations - (L1) 20 forwards, 20 backwards (L2) 20/20 (L3) 20/20
Lateral Body Bends - (L1) 20 to each side (L2) 20/20 (L3) 20/20
Alternate Toe Touches - (L1) 10 to each side (L2) 10/10 (L3) 20/20

Core Training

Roll Backs - (L1) 7 (L2) 9 (L3) 9

Calf Stretches - (L1) 10 (L2) 14 (L3) 15 each leg
Thigh Squeezes - (L1) 10 sets (L2) 10 sets (L3) 10 sets
Full Sit Ups - (L1) 7 (L2) 9 (L3) 18

Cooling Down

Lateral Leans - (L1) 20 each side (L2) 20 each side (L3) 20 each side
Forward Bend & Stretch - (L1) 5 (L2) 5 (L3) 7

Walk up and down for approximately 30 seconds as your pulse rate reduces.
Daily Steps: 10,000 minimum (approximately 5 miles)

WEEK EIGHT

DAY ONE

Limbering Up

Running On The Spot - (L1) 120 seconds (L2) 120 seconds (L3) 120 seconds
Toe Touches - (L1) 20 (L2) 30 (L3) 30
Arm Rotations - (L1) 20 forwards, 20 backwards (L2) 20/20 (L3) 20/20
Lateral Body Bends - (L1) 20 to each side (L2) 20/20 (L3) 20/20
Alternate Toe Touches - (L1) 10 to each side (L2) 10/10 (L3) 20/20

Core Training

Laid Back Kicks - (L1) 16 with each leg (L2) 21 each leg (L3) 40
Lateral Leg Raises - (L1) 16 on each side (L2) 21 each side (L3) 40 each side
Leg Hugs - (L1) 4 (L2) 6 (L3) 13
Pendulum Leg Swings - (L1) 6 (L2) 8 (L3) 18

Cooling Down

Lateral Leans - (L1) 20 each side (L2) 20 each side (L3) 20 each side
Forward Bend & Stretch - (L1) 5 (L2) 5 (L3) 7

Walk up and down for approximately 30 seconds as your pulse rate reduces.
Daily Steps: 10,000 minimum (approximately 5 miles)

DAY TWO

Limbering Up

Running On The Spot – (L1) 120 seconds (L2) 120 seconds (L3) 120 seconds
Toe Touches – (L1) 20 (L2) 30 (L3) 30
Arm Rotations – (L1) 20 forwards, 20 backwards (L2) 20/20 (L3) 20/20
Lateral Body Bends – (L1) 20 to each side (L2) 20/20 (L3) 20/20
Alternate Toe Touches – (L1) 10 to each side (L2) 10/10 (L3) 20/20

Core Training

Laid Back Kicks – (L1) 16 with each leg (L2) 21 each leg (L3) 40
Lateral Leg Raises – (L1) 16 on each side (L2) 21 each side (L3) 40 each side
Leg Hugs – (L1) 5 (L2) 7 (L3) 14
Pendulum Leg Swings – (L1) 6 (L2) 8 (L3) 20

Cooling Down

Lateral Leans – (L1) 20 each side (L2) 20 each side (L3) 20 each side
Forward Bend & Stretch – (L1) 5 (L2) 5 (L3) 7

Walk up and down for approximately 30 seconds as your pulse rate reduces.
Daily Steps: 10,000 minimum (approximately 5 miles)

DAY THREE

Limbering Up

Running On The Spot – (L1) 120 seconds (L2) 120 seconds (L3) 120 seconds
Toe Touches – (L1) 20 (L2) 30 (L3) 30
Arm Rotations – (L1) 20 forwards, 20 backwards (L2) 20/20 (L3) 20/20
Lateral Body Bends – (L1) 20 to each side (L2) 20/20 (L3) 20/20
Alternate Toe Touches – (L1) 10 to each side (L2) 10/10 (L3) 20/20

Core Training

Reverse Curl Ups – (L1) 7 (L2) 9 (L3) 15
Head & Shoulder Lifts – (L1) 9 (L2) 14 (L3) 25

Ab Lifts – (L1) 7 (L2) 8 (L3) 8
Stepped Push Ups (male) – (L1) 7 (L2) 9 (L3) 23 sets
Diamond Push Ups (female) – (L1) 7 (L2) 9 (L3) 15

Cooling Down

Lateral Leans – (L1) 20 each side (L2) 20 each side (L3) 20 each side
Forward Bend & Stretch – (L1) 5 (L2) 5 (L3) 7

Walk up and down for approximately 30 seconds as your pulse rate reduces.
Daily Steps: 10,000 minimum (approximately 5 miles)

DAY FOUR
Limbering Up Only

Running On The Spot – (L1) 120 seconds (L2) 120 seconds (L3) 120 seconds
Toe Touches – (L1) 20 (L2) 30 (L3) 30
Arm Rotations – (L1) 20 forwards, 20 backwards (L2) 20/20 (L3) 20/20
Lateral Body Bends – (L1) 20 to each side (L2) 20/20 (L3) 20/20
Alternate Toe Touches – (L1) 10 to each side (L2) 10/10 (L3) 20/20

Daily Steps: 10,000 minimum (approximately 5 miles)

DAY FIVE
Limbering Up

Running On The Spot – (L1) 120 seconds (L2) 120 seconds (L3) 120 seconds
Toe Touches – (L1) 20 (L2) 30 (L3) 30
Arm Rotations – (L1) 20 forwards, 20 backwards (L2) 20/20 (L3) 20/20
Lateral Body Bends – (L1) 20 to each side (L2) 20/20 (L3) 20/20
Alternate Toe Touches – (L1) 10 to each side (L2) 10/10 (L3) 20/20

Core Training

Reverse Curl Ups – (L1) 8 (L2) 10 (L3) 15
Head & Shoulder Lifts – (L1) 10 (L2) 15 (L3) 25
Ab Lifts – (L1) 7 (L2) 8 (L3) 8
Stepped Push Ups (male) – (L1) 7 (L2) 10 (L3) 25 sets

Diamond Push Ups (female) - (L1) 7 (L2) 10 (L3) 15

Cooling Down

Lateral Leans - (L1) 20 each side (L2) 20 each side (L3) 20 each side
Forward Bend & Stretch - (L1) 5 (L2) 5 (L3) 7

Walk up and down for approximately 30 seconds as your pulse rate reduces.
Daily Steps: 10,000 minimum (approximately 5 miles)

DAY SIX

Limbering Up

Running On The Spot - (L1) 120 seconds (L2) 120 seconds (L3) 120 seconds
Toe Touches - (L1) 20 (L2) 30 (L3) 30
Arm Rotations - (L1) 20 forwards, 20 backwards (L2) 20/20 (L3) 20/20
Lateral Body Bends - (L1) 20 to each side (L2) 20/20 (L3) 20/20
Alternate Toe Touches - (L1) 10 to each side (L2) 10/10 (L3) 20/20

Core Training

Laid Back Kicks - (L1) 17 with each leg (L2) 22 each leg (L3) 40
Lateral Leg Raises - (L1) 17 on each side (L2) 22 each side (L3) 40 each side
Leg Hugs - (L1) 5 (L2) 7 (L3) 15
Pendulum Leg Swings - (L1) 7 (L2) 9 (L3) 20

Cool Down

Lateral Leans - (L1) 20 each side (L2) 20 each side (L3) 20 each side
Forward Bend & Stretch - (L1) 5 (L2) 5 (L3) 7

Walk up and down for approximately 30 seconds as your pulse rate reduces.
Daily Steps: 10,000 minimum (approximately 5 miles)

DAY SEVEN

Limbering Up

Running On The Spot - (L1) 120 seconds (L2) 120 seconds (L3) 120 seconds

Toe Touches – (L1) 20 (L2) 30 (L3) 30
Arm Rotations – (L1) 20 forwards, 20 backwards (L2) 20/20 (L3) 20/20
Lateral Body Bends – (L1) 20 to each side (L2) 20/20 (L3) 20/20
Alternate Toe Touches – (L1) 10 to each side (L2) 10/10 (L3) 20/20

Core Training

Reverse Curl Ups – (L1) 8 (L2) 10 (L3) 15
Head & Shoulder Lifts – (L1) 10 (L2) 15 (L3) 25
Ab Lifts – (L1) 7 (L2) 8 (L3) 8
Stepped Push Ups (male) – (L1) 8 (L2) 10 (L3) 27 sets
Diamond Push Ups (female) – (L1) 8 (L2) 10 (L3) 15

Cooling Down

Lateral Leans – (L1) 20 each side (L2) 20 each side (L3) 20 each side
Forward Bend & Stretch – (L1) 5 (L2) 5 (L3) 7

Walk up and down for approximately 30 seconds as your pulse rate reduces.
Daily Steps: 10,000 minimum (approximately 5 miles)

Eight Weeks completed. You should be feeling considerably fitter by now, even though there is plenty of room for improvement. Well done for persisting. Now it is time to for a final push towards your 12 Week Goal. Review your Weekly Targets once again. Still achieving an 85% strike rate - about 6 days out of 7? Think deeply about your main vision, your long-term goal, and re-set your targets to ensure that it doesn't remain just a pipe dream.

Have you been sticking with the main Exercise Plan? You should have been completing at least an 85% strike rate, and preferably 100% if you are to reap the full rewards. Now there are just 4 weeks left in the initial 12-Week Plan for your greater fitness and you should be fit enough to exercise every day to take it to the max.

WEEK NINE

DAY ONE

Limbering Up

Running On The Spot - (L1) 120 seconds (L2) 120 seconds (L3) 120 seconds
Toe Touches - (L1) 20 (L2) 30 (L3) 30
Arm Rotations - (L1) 20 forwards, 20 backwards (L2) 20/20 (L3) 20/20
Lateral Body Bends - (L1) 20 to each side (L2) 20/20 (L3) 20/20
Alternate Toe Touches - (L1) 10 to each side (L2) 10/10 (L3) 20/20

Core Training

Abdominal Strength Training - (L1) 10 (L2) 12 (L3) 20
Hand to Foot - (L1) 9 (L2) 14 (L3) 20
Arm Lifts - (L1) 16 (5 Left, 5 Right, 6 together) (L2) 21 (7/7/7) (L3) 36 (12/12/12)
Full Sit Ups - (L1) 7 (L2) 9 (L3) 19

Cooling Down

Lateral Leans - (L1) 20 each side (L2) 20 each side (L3) 20 each side
Forward Bend & Stretch - (L1) 5 (L2) 5 (L3) 7

Walk up and down for approximately 30 seconds as your pulse rate reduces.
Daily Steps: 10,000 minimum (approximately 5 miles)

DAY TWO

Limbering Up

Running On The Spot - (L1) 120 seconds (L2) 120 seconds (L3) 120 seconds
Toe Touches - (L1) 20 (L2) 30 (L3) 30
Arm Rotations - (L1) 20 forwards, 20 backwards (L2) 20/20 (L3) 20/20
Lateral Body Bends - (L1) 20 to each side (L2) 20/20 (L3) 20/20
Alternate Toe Touches - (L1) 10 to each side (L2) 10/10 (L3) 20/20

Core Training

Abdominal Strength Training - (L1) 11 (L2) 13 (L3) 20

Hand to Foot – (L1) 10 (L2) 15 (L3) 20
Arm Lifts – (L1) 16 (5 Left, 5 Right, 6 together) (L2) 21 (7/7/7) (L3) 36 (12/12/12)
Full Sit Ups – (L1) 8 (L2) 10 (L3) 20

Cooling Down

Lateral Leans – (L1) 20 each side (L2) 20 each side (L3) 20 each side
Forward Bend & Stretch – (L1) 5 (L2) 5 (L3) 7

Walk up and down for approximately 30 seconds as your pulse rate reduces.
Daily Steps: 10,000 minimum (approximately 5 miles)

DAY THREE

Limbering Up

Running On The Spot – (L1) 120 seconds (L2) 120 seconds (L3) 120 seconds
Toe Touches – (L1) 20 (L2) 30 (L3) 30
Arm Rotations – (L1) 20 forwards, 20 backwards (L2) 20/20 (L3) 20/20
Lateral Body Bends – (L1) 20 to each side (L2) 20/20 (L3) 20/20
Alternate Toe Touches – (L1) 10 to each side (L2) 10/10 (L3) 20/20

Core Training

Leg-Passing Knee Pulls – (L1) 9 (L2) 11 (L3) 15
Thigh Squeezes – (L1) 10 sets (L2) 10 sets (L3) 10 sets
Roll Backs – (L1) 7 (L2) 9 (L3) 9
Leg Hugs – (L1) 6 (L2) 8 (L3) 16

Cooling Down

Lateral Leans – (L1) 20 each side (L2) 20 each side (L3) 20 each side
Forward Bend & Stretch – (L1) 5 (L2) 5 (L3) 7

Walk up and down for approximately 30 seconds as your pulse rate reduces.
Daily Steps: 10,000 minimum (approximately 5 miles)

DAY FOUR

Limbering Up

Running On The Spot - (L1) 120 seconds (L2) 120 seconds (L3) 120 seconds
Toe Touches - (L1) 20 (L2) 30 (L3) 30
Arm Rotations - (L1) 20 forwards, 20 backwards (L2) 20/20 (L3) 20/20
Lateral Body Bends - (L1) 20 to each side (L2) 20/20 (L3) 20/20
Alternate Toe Touches - (L1) 10 to each side (L2) 10/10 (L3) 20/20

Core Training

Leg-Passing Knee Pulls - (L1) 9 (L2) 11 (L3) 15
Thigh Squeezes - (L1) 10 sets (L2) 10 sets (L3) 10 sets
Roll Backs - (L1) 7 (L2) 9 (L3) 9
Leg Hugs - (L1) 6 (L2) 8 (L3) 18

Cooling Down

Lateral Leans - (L1) 20 each side (L2) 20 each side (L3) 20 each side
Forward Bend & Stretch - (L1) 5 (L2) 5 (L3) 7

Walk up and down for approximately 30 seconds as your pulse rate reduces.
Daily Steps: 10,000 minimum (approximately 5 miles)

DAY FIVE

Limbering Up

Running On The Spot - (L1) 120 seconds (L2) 120 seconds (L3) 120 seconds
Toe Touches - (L1) 20 (L2) 30 (L3) 30
Arm Rotations - (L1) 20 forwards, 20 backwards (L2) 20/20 (L3) 20/20
Lateral Body Bends - (L1) 20 to each side (L2) 20/20 (L3) 20/20
Alternate Toe Touches - (L1) 10 to each side (L2) 10/10 (L3) 20/20

Core Training

Abdominal Strength Training - (L1) 11 (L2) 13 (L3) 20
Hand to Foot - (L1) 10 (L2) 15 (L3) 20
Arm Lifts - (L1) 17 (5 Left, 5 Right, 7 together) (L2) 22 (7/7/8) (L3) 36 (12/12/12)
Full Sit Ups - (L1) 8 (L2) 10 (L3) 22

Cooling Down

Lateral Leans – (L1) 20 each side (L2) 20 each side (L3) 20 each side
Forward Bend & Stretch – (L1) 5 (L2) 5 (L3) 7

Walk up and down for approximately 30 seconds as your pulse rate reduces.
Daily Steps: 10,000 minimum (approximately 5 miles)

DAY SIX

Limbering Up

Running On The Spot – (L1) 120 seconds (L2) 120 seconds (L3) 120 seconds
Toe Touches – (L1) 20 (L2) 30 (L3) 30
Arm Rotations – (L1) 20 forwards, 20 backwards (L2) 20/20 (L3) 20/20
Lateral Body Bends – (L1) 20 to each side (L2) 20/20 (L3) 20/20
Alternate Toe Touches – (L1) 10 to each side (L2) 10/10 (L3) 20/20

Core Training

Leg-Passing Knee Pulls – (L1) 10 (L2) 12 (L3) 15
Thigh Squeezes – (L1) 10 sets (L2) 10 sets (L3) 10 sets
Roll Backs – (L1) 7 (L2) 9 (L3) 9
Leg Hugs – (L1) 7 (L2) 9 (L3) 20

Cooling Down

Lateral Leans – (L1) 20 each side (L2) 20 each side (L3) 20 each side
Forward Bend & Stretch – (L1) 5 (L2) 5 (L3) 7

Walk up and down for approximately 30 seconds as your pulse rate reduces.
Daily Steps: 10,000 minimum (approximately 5 miles)

DAY SEVEN

Limbering Up

Running On The Spot – (L1) 120 seconds (L2) 120 seconds (L3) 120 seconds
Toe Touches – (L1) 20 (L2) 30 (L3) 30
Arm Rotations – (L1) 20 forwards, 20 backwards (L2) 20/20 (L3) 20/20

Lateral Body Bends - (L1) 20 to each side (L2) 20/20 (L3) 20/20
Alternate Toe Touches - (L1) 10 to each side (L2) 10/10 (L3) 20/20

Core Training

Abdominal Strength Training - (L1) 12 (L2) 14 (L3) 20
Hand to Foot - (L1) 11 (L2) 16 (L3) 20
Arm Lifts - (L1) 17 (5 Left, 5 Right, 7 together) (L2) 22 (7/7/8) (L3) 36 (12/12/12)
Full Sit Ups - (L1) 9 (L2) 11 (L3) 24

Cooling Down

Lateral Leans - (L1) 20 each side (L2) 20 each side (L3) 20 each side
Forward Bend & Stretch - (L1) 5 (L2) 5 (L3) 7

Walk up and down for approximately 30 seconds as your pulse rate reduces.
Daily Steps: 10,000 minimum (approximately 5 miles)

WEEK TEN

DAY ONE

Limbering Up

Running On The Spot - (L1) 120 seconds (L2) 120 seconds (L3) 120 seconds
Toe Touches - (L1) 20 (L2) 30 (L3) 30
Arm Rotations - (L1) 20 forwards, 20 backwards (L2) 20/20 (L3) 20/20
Lateral Body Bends - (L1) 20 to each side (L2) 20/20 (L3) 20/20
Alternate Toe Touches - (L1) 10 to each side (L2) 10/10 (L3) 20/20

Core Training

Laid Back Kicks - (L1) 17 with each leg (L2) 22 each leg (L3) 40
Head & Shoulder Lifts - (L1) 11 (L2) 16 (L3) 25
Calf Stretches - (L1) 10 (L2) 14 (L3) 15
Stepped Push Ups (male) - (L1) 8 (L2) 11 (L3) 29 sets
Diamond Push Ups (female) - (L1) 8 (L2) 11 (L3) 15

Cooling Down

Lateral Leans – (L1) 20 each side (L2) 20 each side (L3) 20 each side
Forward Bend & Stretch – (L1) 5 (L2) 5 (L3) 7

Walk up and down for approximately 30 seconds as your pulse rate reduces.
Daily Steps: 10,000 minimum (approximately 5 miles)

DAY TWO

Limbering Up

Running On The Spot – (L1) 120 seconds (L2) 120 seconds (L3) 120 seconds
Toe Touches – (L1) 20 (L2) 30 (L3) 30
Arm Rotations – (L1) 20 forwards, 20 backwards (L2) 20/20 (L3) 20/20
Lateral Body Bends – (L1) 20 to each side (L2) 20/20 (L3) 20/20
Alternate Toe Touches – (L1) 10 to each side (L2) 10/10 (L3) 20/20

Core Training

Laid Back Kicks – (L1) 18 with each leg (L2) 23 each leg (L3) 40
Head & Shoulder Lifts – (L1) 11 (L2) 16 (L3) 25
Calf Stretches – (L1) 10 (L2) 15 (L3) 15
Stepped Push Ups (male) – (L1) 9 (L2) 11 (L3) 30 sets
Diamond Push Ups (female) – (L1) 9 (L2) 11 (L3) 15

Cooling Down

Lateral Leans – (L1) 20 each side (L2) 20 each side (L3) 20 each side
Forward Bend & Stretch – (L1) 5 (L2) 5 (L3) 7

Walk up and down for approximately 30 seconds as your pulse rate reduces.
Daily Steps: 10,000 minimum (approximately 5 miles)

DAY THREE

Limbering Up

Running On The Spot – (L1) 120 seconds (L2) 120 seconds (L3) 120 seconds
Toe Touches – (L1) 20 (L2) 30 (L3) 30

Arm Rotations – (L1) 20 forwards, 20 backwards (L2) 20/20 (L3) 20/20
Lateral Body Bends – (L1) 20 to each side (L2) 20/20 (L3) 20/20
Alternate Toe Touches – (L1) 10 to each side (L2) 10/10 (L3) 20/20

Core Training

Abdominal Strength Training – (L1) 12 (L2) 14 (L3) 20
Reverse Curl Ups – (L1) 9 (L2) 11 (L3) 15
Lateral Leg Raises – (L1) 17 on each side (L2) 22 each side (L3) 40 each side
Pendulum Leg Swings – (L1) 7 (L2) 9 (L3) 20

Cooling Down

Lateral Leans – (L1) 20 each side (L2) 20 each side (L3) 20 each side
Forward Bend & Stretch – (L1) 5 (L2) 5 (L3) 7

Walk up and down for approximately 30 seconds as your pulse rate reduces.
Daily Steps: 10,000 minimum (approximately 5 miles)

DAY FOUR
Limbering Up

Running On The Spot – (L1) 120 seconds (L2) 120 seconds (L3) 120 seconds
Toe Touches – (L1) 20 (L2) 30 (L3) 30
Arm Rotations – (L1) 20 forwards, 20 backwards (L2) 20/20 (L3) 20/20
Lateral Body Bends – (L1) 20 to each side (L2) 20/20 (L3) 20/20
Alternate Toe Touches – (L1) 10 to each side (L2) 10/10 (L3) 20/20

Core Training

Abdominal Strength Training – (L1) 13 (L2) 15 (L3) 20
Reverse Curl Ups – (L1) 9 (L2) 11 (L3) 15
Lateral Leg Raises – (L1) 18 on each side (L2) 23 each side (L3) 40 each side
Pendulum Leg Swings – (L1) 8 (L2) 10 (L3) 20

Cooling Down

Lateral Leans – (L1) 20 each side (L2) 20 each side (L3) 20 each side
Forward Bend & Stretch – (L1) 5 (L2) 5 (L3) 7

Walk up and down for approximately 30 seconds as your pulse rate reduces.
Daily Steps: 10,000 minimum (approximately 5 miles)

DAY FIVE

Limbering Up

Running On The Spot - (L1) 120 seconds (L2) 120 seconds (L3) 120 seconds
Toe Touches - (L1) 20 (L2) 30 (L3) 30
Arm Rotations - (L1) 20 forwards, 20 backwards (L2) 20/20 (L3) 20/20
Lateral Body Bends - (L1) 20 to each side (L2) 20/20 (L3) 20/20
Alternate Toe Touches - (L1) 10 to each side (L2) 10/10 (L3) 20/20

Core Training

Laid Back Kicks - (L1) 18 with each leg (L2) 23 each leg (L3) 40
Head & Shoulder Lifts - (L1) 12 (L2) 17 (L3) 25
Calf Stretches - (L1) 10 (L2) 15 (L3) 15
Stepped Push Ups (male) - (L1) 9 (L2) 12 (L3) 30 sets
Diamond Push Ups (female) - (L1) 9 (L2) 12 (L3) 15

Cooling Down

Lateral Leans - (L1) 20 each side (L2) 20 each side (L3) 20 each side
Forward Bend & Stretch - (L1) 5 (L2) 5 (L3) 7

Walk up and down for approximately 30 seconds as your pulse rate reduces.
Daily Steps: 10,000 minimum (approximately 5 miles)

DAY SIX

Limbering Up

Running On The Spot - (L1) 120 seconds (L2) 120 seconds (L3) 120 seconds
Toe Touches - (L1) 20 (L2) 30 (L3) 30
Arm Rotations - (L1) 20 forwards, 20 backwards (L2) 20/20 (L3) 20/20
Lateral Body Bends - (L1) 20 to each side (L2) 20/20 (L3) 20/20
Alternate Toe Touches - (L1) 10 to each side (L2) 10/10 (L3) 20/20

Core Training

Abdominal Strength Training - (L1) 13 (L2) 15 (L3) 20
Reverse Curl Ups - (L1) 10 (L2) 12 (L3) 15
Lateral Leg Raises - (L1) 18 on each side (L2) 23 each side (L3) 40 each side
Pendulum Leg Swings - (L1) 8 (L2) 10 (L3) 20

Cooling Down

Lateral Leans - (L1) 20 each side (L2) 20 each side (L3) 20 each side
Forward Bend & Stretch - (L1) 5 (L2) 5 (L3) 7

Walk up and down for approximately 30 seconds as your pulse rate reduces.
Daily Steps: 10,000 minimum (approximately 5 miles)

DAY SEVEN

Limbering Up

Running On The Spot - (L1) 120 seconds (L2) 120 seconds (L3) 120 seconds
Toe Touches - (L1) 20 (L2) 30 (L3) 30
Arm Rotations - (L1) 20 forwards, 20 backwards (L2) 20/20 (L3) 20/20
Lateral Body Bends - (L1) 20 to each side (L2) 20/20 (L3) 20/20
Alternate Toe Touches - (L1) 10 to each side (L2) 10/10 (L3) 20/20

Core Training

Laid Back Kicks - (L1) 19 with each leg (L2) 24 each leg (L3) 40
Head & Shoulder Lifts - (L1) 12 (L2) 17 (L3) 25
Calf Stretches - (L1) 10 (L2) 15 (L3) 15
Stepped Push Ups (male) - (L1) 10 (L2) 12 (L3) 30 sets
Diamond Push Ups (female) - (L1) 10 (L2) 12 (L3) 15

Cooling Down

Lateral Leans - (L1) 20 each side (L2) 20 each side (L3) 20 each side
Forward Bend & Stretch - (L1) 5 (L2) 5 (L3) 7

Walk up and down for approximately 30 seconds as your pulse rate reduces.
Daily Steps: 10,000 minimum (approximately 5 miles)

WEEK ELEVEN

DAY ONE

Limbering Up

Running On The Spot – (L1) 120 seconds (L2) 120 seconds (L3) 120 seconds
Toe Touches – (L1) 20 (L2) 30 (L3) 30
Arm Rotations – (L1) 20 forwards, 20 backwards (L2) 20/20 (L3) 20/20
Lateral Body Bends – (L1) 20 to each side (L2) 20/20 (L3) 20/20
Alternate Toe Touches – (L1) 10 to each side (L2) 10/10 (L3) 20/20

Core Training

Roll Backs – (L1) 7 (L2) 9 (L3) 9
Leg Hugs – (L1) 7 (L2) 9 (L3) 20
Arm Lifts – (L1) 18 (6 Left, 6 Right, 6 together) (L2) 23 (7/7/9) (L3) 36 (12/12/12)
Stepped Push Ups (male) – (L1) 10 (L2) 13 (L3) 30 sets
Diamond Push Ups (female) – (L1) 10 (L2) 13 (L3) 15

Cooling Down

Lateral Leans – (L1) 20 each side (L2) 20 each side (L3) 20 each side
Forward Bend & Stretch – (L1) 5 (L2) 5 (L3) 7

Walk up and down for approximately 30 seconds as your pulse rate reduces.
Daily Steps: 10,000 minimum (approximately 5 miles)

DAY TWO

Limbering Up

Running On The Spot – (L1) 120 seconds (L2) 120 seconds (L3) 120 seconds
Toe Touches – (L1) 20 (L2) 30 (L3) 30
Arm Rotations – (L1) 20 forwards, 20 backwards (L2) 20/20 (L3) 20/20
Lateral Body Bends – (L1) 20 to each side (L2) 20/20 (L3) 20/20
Alternate Toe Touches – (L1) 10 to each side (L2) 10/10 (L3) 20/20

Core Training

Roll Backs - (L1) 7 (L2) 9 (L3) 9
Leg Hugs - (L1) 8 (L2) 10 (L3) 20
Arm Lifts - (L1) 18 (6 Left, 6 Right, 6 together) (L2) 23 (7/7/9) (L3) 36 (12/12/12)
Stepped Push Ups (male) – (L1) 11 (L2) 13 (L3) 30 sets
Diamond Push Ups (female) - (L1) 11 (L2) 13 (L3) 15

Cooling Down

Lateral Leans - (L1) 20 each side (L2) 20 each side (L3) 20 each side
Forward Bend & Stretch - (L1) 5 (L2) 5 (L3) 7

Walk up and down for approximately 30 seconds as your pulse rate reduces.
Daily Steps: 10,000 minimum (approximately 5 miles)

DAY THREE

Limbering Up

Running On The Spot - (L1) 120 seconds (L2) 120 seconds (L3) 120 seconds
Toe Touches - (L1) 20 (L2) 30 (L3) 30
Arm Rotations - (L1) 20 forwards, 20 backwards (L2) 20/20 (L3) 20/20
Lateral Body Bends - (L1) 20 to each side (L2) 20/20 (L3) 20/20
Alternate Toe Touches - (L1) 10 to each side (L2) 10/10 (L3) 20/20

Core Training

Laid Back Kicks - (L1) 19 with each leg (L2) 24 each leg (L3) 40
Hand to Foot - (L1) 11 (L2) 16 (L3) 20
Ab Lifts - (L1) 7 (L2) 8 (L3) 8
Full Sit Ups – (L1) 9 (L2) 11 (L3) 26

Cooling Down

Lateral Leans - (L1) 20 each side (L2) 20 each side (L3) 20 each side
Forward Bend & Stretch - (L1) 5 (L2) 5 (L3) 7

Walk up and down for approximately 30 seconds as your pulse rate reduces.
Daily Steps: 10,000 minimum (approximately 5 miles)

DAY FOUR

Limbering Up

Running On The Spot – (L1) 120 seconds (L2) 120 seconds (L3) 120 seconds
Toe Touches – (L1) 20 (L2) 30 (L3) 30
Arm Rotations – (L1) 20 forwards, 20 backwards (L2) 20/20 (L3) 20/20
Lateral Body Bends – (L1) 20 to each side (L2) 20/20 (L3) 20/20
Alternate Toe Touches – (L1) 10 to each side (L2) 10/10 (L3) 20/20

Core Training

Laid Back Kicks – (L1) 20 with each leg (L2) 25 each leg (L3) 40
Hand to Foot – (L1) 12 (L2) 17 (L3) 20
Ab Lifts – (L1) 7 (L2) 8 (L3) 8
Full Sit Ups – (L1) 10 (L2) 12 (L3) 28

Cooling Down

Lateral Leans – (L1) 20 each side (L2) 20 each side (L3) 20 each side
Forward Bend & Stretch – (L1) 5 (L2) 5 (L3) 7

Walk up and down for approximately 30 seconds as your pulse rate reduces.
Daily Steps: 10,000 minimum (approximately 5 miles)

DAY FIVE

Limbering Up

Running On The Spot – (L1) 120 seconds (L2) 120 seconds (L3) 120 seconds
Toe Touches – (L1) 20 (L2) 30 (L3) 30
Arm Rotations – (L1) 20 forwards, 20 backwards (L2) 20/20 (L3) 20/20
Lateral Body Bends – (L1) 20 to each side (L2) 20/20 (L3) 20/20
Alternate Toe Touches – (L1) 10 to each side (L2) 10/10 (L3) 20/20

Core Training

Roll Backs – (L1) 7 (L2) 9 (L3) 9
Leg Hugs – (L1) 8 (L2) 10 (L3) 20

Arm Lifts - (L1) 19 (6 Left, 6 Right, 7 together) (L2) 24 (8/8/8) (L3) 36 (12/12/12)
Stepped Push Ups (male) - (L1) 11 (L2) 14 (L3) 30 sets
Diamond Push Ups (female) - (L1) 11 (L2) 14 (L3) 15

Cooling Down

Lateral Leans - (L1) 20 each side (L2) 20 each side (L3) 20 each side
Forward Bend & Stretch - (L1) 5 (L2) 5 (L3) 7

Walk up and down for approximately 30 seconds as your pulse rate reduces.
Daily Steps: 10,000 minimum (approximately 5 miles)

DAY SIX

Limbering Up

Running On The Spot - (L1) 120 seconds (L2) 120 seconds (L3) 120 seconds
Toe Touches - (L1) 20 (L2) 30 (L3) 30
Arm Rotations - (L1) 20 forwards, 20 backwards (L2) 20/20 (L3) 20/20
Lateral Body Bends - (L1) 20 to each side (L2) 20/20 (L3) 20/20
Alternate Toe Touches - (L1) 10 to each side (L2) 10/10 (L3) 20/20

Core Training

Laid Back Kicks - (L1) 20 with each leg (L2) 25 each leg (L3) 40
Hand to Foot - (L1) 12 (L2) 17 (L3) 20
Ab Lifts - (L1) 7 (L2) 8 (L3) 8
Full Sit Ups - (L1) 10 (L2) 12 (L3) 30

Cooling Down

Lateral Leans - (L1) 20 each side (L2) 20 each side (L3) 20 each side
Forward Bend & Stretch - (L1) 5 (L2) 5 (L3) 7

Walk up and down for approximately 30 seconds as your pulse rate reduces.
Daily Steps: 10,000 minimum (approximately 5 miles)

DAY SEVEN

Limbering Up

Running On The Spot – (L1) 120 seconds (L2) 120 seconds (L3) 120 seconds
Toe Touches – (L1) 20 (L2) 30 (L3) 30
Arm Rotations – (L1) 20 forwards, 20 backwards (L2) 20/20 (L3) 20/20
Lateral Body Bends – (L1) 20 to each side (L2) 20/20 (L3) 20/20
Alternate Toe Touches – (L1) 10 to each side (L2) 10/10 (L3) 20/20

Core Training

Roll Backs – (L1) 7 (L2) 9 (L3) 9
Leg Hugs – (L1) 9 (L2) 11 (L3) 20
Arm Lifts – (L1) 19 (6 Left, 6 Right, 7 together) (L2) 24 (8/8/8) (L3) 36 (12/12/12)
Stepped Push Ups (male) – (L1) 12 (L2) 14 (L3) 30 sets
Diamond Push Ups (female) – (L1) 12 (L2) 14 (L3) 15

Cooling Down

Lateral Leans – (L1) 20 each side (L2) 20 each side (L3) 20 each side
Forward Bend & Stretch – (L1) 5 (L2) 5 (L3) 7

Walk up and down for approximately 30 seconds as your pulse rate reduces.
Daily Steps: 10,000 minimum (approximately 5 miles)

WEEK TWELVE

DAY ONE

Limbering Up

Running On The Spot – (L1) 120 seconds (L2) 120 seconds (L3) 120 seconds
Toe Touches – (L1) 20 (L2) 30 (L3) 30
Arm Rotations – (L1) 20 forwards, 20 backwards (L2) 20/20 (L3) 20/20
Lateral Body Bends – (L1) 20 to each side (L2) 20/20 (L3) 20/20
Alternate Toe Touches – (L1) 10 to each side (L2) 10/10 (L3) 20/20

Core Training

Leg–Passing Knee Pulls – (L1) 10 (L2) 12 (L3) 15
Pendulum Leg Swings – (L1) 9 (L2) 11 (L3) 20

Head & Shoulder Lifts - (L1) 13 (L2) 18 (L3) 25
Thigh Squeezes - (L1) 10 sets (L2) 10 sets (L3) 10 sets

Cooling Down

Lateral Leans - (L1) 20 each side (L2) 20 each side (L3) 20 each side
Forward Bend & Stretch - (L1) 5 (L2) 5 (L3) 7

Walk up and down for approximately 30 seconds as your pulse rate reduces.
Daily Steps: 10,000 minimum (approximately 5 miles)

DAY TWO

Limbering Up

Running On The Spot - (L1) 120 seconds (L2) 120 seconds (L3) 120 seconds
Toe Touches - (L1) 20 (L2) 30 (L3) 30
Arm Rotations - (L1) 20 forwards, 20 backwards (L2) 20/20 (L3) 20/20
Lateral Body Bends - (L1) 20 to each side (L2) 20/20 (L3) 20/20
Alternate Toe Touches - (L1) 10 to each side (L2) 10/10 (L3) 20/20

Core Training

Leg-Passing Knee Pulls - (L1) 11 (L2) 13 (L3) 15
Pendulum Leg Swings - (L1) 9 (L2) 11 (L3) 20
Head & Shoulder Lifts - (L1) 13 (L2) 18 (L3) 25
Thigh Squeezes - (L1) 10 sets (L2) 10 sets (L3) 10 sets

Cooling Down

Lateral Leans - (L1) 20 each side (L2) 20 each side (L3) 20 each side
Forward Bend & Stretch - (L1) 5 (L2) 5 (L3) 7

Walk up and down for approximately 30 seconds as your pulse rate reduces.
Daily Steps: 10,000 minimum (approximately 5 miles)

DAY THREE

Limbering Up

Running On The Spot – (L1) 120 seconds (L2) 120 seconds (L3) 120 seconds
Toe Touches – (L1) 20 (L2) 30 (L3) 30
Arm Rotations – (L1) 20 forwards, 20 backwards (L2) 20/20 (L3) 20/20
Lateral Body Bends – (L1) 20 to each side (L2) 20/20 (L3) 20/20
Alternate Toe Touches – (L1) 10 to each side (L2) 10/10 (L3) 20/20

Core Training

Abdominal Strength Training – (L1) 14 (L2) 16 (L3) 20
Roll Backs – (L1) 7 (L2) 9 (L3) 9
Arm Lifts – (L1) 20 (6 Left, 6 Right, 8 together) (L2) 25 (8/8/9) (L3) 36 (12/12/12)
Leg Hugs – (L1) 9 (L2) 11 (L3) 20

Cooling Down

Lateral Leans – (L1) 20 each side (L2) 20 each side (L3) 20 each side
Forward Bend & Stretch – (L1) 5 (L2) 5 (L3) 7

Walk up and down for approximately 30 seconds as your pulse rate reduces.
Daily Steps: 10,000 minimum (approximately 5 miles)

DAY FOUR

Limbering Up

Running On The Spot – (L1) 120 seconds (L2) 120 seconds (L3) 120 seconds
Toe Touches – (L1) 20 (L2) 30 (L3) 30
Arm Rotations – (L1) 20 forwards, 20 backwards (L2) 20/20 (L3) 20/20
Lateral Body Bends – (L1) 20 to each side (L2) 20/20 (L3) 20/20
Alternate Toe Touches – (L1) 10 to each side (L2) 10/10 (L3) 20/20

Core Training

Abdominal Strength Training – (L1) 14 (L2) 16 (L3) 20
Roll Backs – (L1) 7 (L2) 9 (L3) 9
Arm Lifts – (L1) 20 (6 Left, 6 Right, 8 together) (L2) 25 (8/8/9) (L3) 36 (12/12/12)
Leg Hugs – (L1) 10 (L2) 12 (L3) 20

Cooling Down

Lateral Leans - (L1) 20 each side (L2) 20 each side (L3) 20 each side
Forward Bend & Stretch - (L1) 5 (L2) 5 (L3) 7

Walk up and down for approximately 30 seconds as your pulse rate reduces.
Daily Steps: 10,000 minimum (approximately 5 miles)

DAY FIVE

Limbering Up

Running On The Spot - (L1) 120 seconds (L2) 120 seconds (L3) 120 seconds
Toe Touches - (L1) 20 (L2) 30 (L3) 30
Arm Rotations - (L1) 20 forwards, 20 backwards (L2) 20/20 (L3) 20/20
Lateral Body Bends - (L1) 20 to each side (L2) 20/20 (L3) 20/20
Alternate Toe Touches - (L1) 10 to each side (L2) 10/10 (L3) 20/20

Core Training

Leg-Passing Knee Pulls - (L1) 11 (L2) 13 (L3) 15
Pendulum Leg Swings - (L1) 10 (L2) 12 (L3) 20
Head & Shoulder Lifts - (L1) 14 (L2) 19 (L3) 25
Thigh Squeezes - (L1) 10 sets (L2) 10 sets (L3) 10 sets

Cooling Down

Lateral Leans - (L1) 20 each side (L2) 20 each side (L3) 20 each side
Forward Bend & Stretch - (L1) 5 (L2) 5 (L3) 7

Walk up and down for approximately 30 seconds as your pulse rate reduces.
Daily Steps: 10,000 minimum (approximately 5 miles)

DAY SIX

Limbering Up

Running On The Spot - (L1) 120 seconds (L2) 120 seconds (L3) 120 seconds
Toe Touches - (L1) 20 (L2) 30 (L3) 30
Arm Rotations - (L1) 20 forwards, 20 backwards (L2) 20/20 (L3) 20/20
Lateral Body Bends - (L1) 20 to each side (L2) 20/20 (L3) 20/20
Alternate Toe Touches - (L1) 10 to each side (L2) 10/10 (L3) 20/20

Core Training

Abdominal Strength Training – (L1) 15 (L2) 16 (L3) 20
Roll Backs – (L1) 7 (L2) 9 (L3) 9
Arm Lifts – (L1) 21 (7 Left, 7 Right, 7 together) (L2) 26 (8/8/10) (L3) 36 (12/12/12)
Leg Hugs – (L1) 10 (L2) 12 (L3) 20

Cooling Down

Lateral Leans – (L1) 20 each side (L2) 20 each side (L3) 20 each side
Forward Bend & Stretch – (L1) 5 (L2) 5 (L3) 7

Walk up and down for approximately 30 seconds as your pulse rate reduces.
Daily Steps: 10,000 minimum (approximately 5 miles)

DAY SEVEN

Limbering Up

Running On The Spot – (L1) 120 seconds (L2) 120 seconds (L3) 120 seconds
Toe Touches – (L1) 20 (L2) 30 (L3) 30
Arm Rotations – (L1) 20 forwards, 20 backwards (L2) 20/20 (L3) 20/20
Lateral Body Bends – (L1) 20 to each side (L2) 20/20 (L3) 20/20
Alternate Toe Touches – (L1) 10 to each side (L2) 10/10 (L3) 20/20

Core Training

Leg-Passing Knee Pulls – (L1) 12 (L2) 14 (L3) 15
Pendulum Leg Swings – (L1) 10 (L2) 12 (L3) 20
Head & Shoulder Lifts – (L1) 14 (L2) 19 (L3) 25
Thigh Squeezes – (L1) 10 sets (L2) 10 sets (L3) 10 sets

Cooling Down

Lateral Leans – (L1) 20 each side (L2) 20 each side (L3) 20 each side
Forward Bend & Stretch – (L1) 5 (L2) 5 (L3) 7

Walk up and down for approximately 30 seconds as your pulse rate reduces.
Daily Steps: 10,000 minimum (approximately 5 miles)

IS THIS THE END?

Congratulations. You have completed your Twelve Week program! Have you achieved all that you set out to accomplish? What improvements have you made? Whether it is a trimmer waistline, general weight loss, or a welcome feeling of greater fitness, I would be delighted to know what has improved for you so far. If you have achieved your initial target, or made great strides in that direction then please let me know. If you are disappointed with your results then also let me know. Your feedback is important.

I hope that you have made amazing progress during the last 12 weeks and that you are inspired to continue. Now that you have mastered all the exercises in the 12 Week Exercise Plan, there is no reason to stop now. You have accessed the keys to a fitter future. You have taken it for a test drive. Now you own your future.

Your chosen Diet Plan can be used as a framework for your dietary health, but there is no need to stick rigidly to a plan which is designed for active weight loss. The essence of either plan amounts to 'Clean Eating', which you can learn more about at https://easyfitnessfor life.net

So where do you go from here?

Think back to your Vision, your grand plan for where you want to be in the future. You have just progressed 12 weeks closer to it, positively and in charge of your future.

Now is a good time to step back and consider your main target for the coming 12 weeks. Make this day a Rest Day, even two, after your boosted efforts over the last four weeks, and think about setting a new challenging target to reach 12 weeks from now. Then, as before, you can set out some new weekly targets which will help you to get there.

Continue with exactly the same sequence of exercises, incorporating a rest day one day a week except for those occasions when you feel the need for an extra push. On the next page you will find a guide to the maximum recommended level for each exercise – which I term The Maintenance Level - to maintain your fitness now and far into the future. Those on the Level Three plan will already have reached these highs and should have no difficulty in continuing. Anyone following the Level One or Level Two plans may progress to the maximum, gradually, *until you feel capable of it.*

The Maintenance Level

Alternate Toe Touches - 20 to each side
Arm Rotations - 20 forwards, 20 backwards
Lateral Body Bends - 20 to each side
Running On The Spot - 120 seconds
Toe Touches - 30

Ab Lifts – 8
Abdominal Strength Training – 20
Arm Lifts – 36 with each arm
Calf Stretches - 15
Full Sit Ups – 30
Hand and Foot - 20
Head & Shoulder Lifts - 25
Laid Back Kicks - 40 with each leg
Lateral Leg Raises - 40 with each leg
Leg Hugs – 20 with each leg
Leg-Passing Knee Pulls – 15
Pendulum Leg Swings - 20
Stepped Push Ups (male) - 30
Diamond Push Ups (female) - 15
Reverse Curl Ups - 15
Roll Backs – 9
Thigh Squeezes - 10 sets

Forward Bend & Stretch – 7
Lateral Leans - 20 each side

When you have reached this Maintenance Level then your future fitness should be assured. Even if you miss a day or two of these routine exercises every now and then. Even if you succumb to spells of excessive over-indulgence at certain times of the year. That shouldn't be a problem.

Bear in mind, however, that although your fitness won't desert you without some serious neglect on your part, it will become increasingly difficult to regain it after a few weeks without proper exercise. Every now and then you may gain a few pounds if you have over-indulged just that bit too much. This will be quite easy to shed after a few days of a lower calorie intake, equivalent to whatever led to the excess, in addition to extra exercise over and above the maintenance level.

Be careful though. The longer the period of neglecting your fitness the easier it becomes to put off the day when you pick it up again. Not only that, but you will be discouraged by the difficulty of resuming any exercise routines. Please don't allow that to happen now that you have come this far.

Easy Fitness is easy. It only becomes more challenging when you let your fitness level fall. You really don't want to start again with Week One after years of inactivity. Trust me, I know!

Now that you have completed your first 12 weeks of exercise, you are well set for a better, fitter, future. However, you don't need to go there alone. Let me help you maintain that fitness level, encourage you to continue when your resolve may be weakening, and even show you how to progress to another level. You have taken the right path towards a much healthier lifestyle, and I hope you will agree that setting out on this journey and arriving at this milestone post has been much easier than you first thought.

If you would like to join me in the *Easy Fitness* group then we can continue on this journey together. This is the end of the book, but it need not stop right here.

Remember, as you grow older your muscles start wasting away – if you don't use them. So keep it up, and if you need support in continuing your progress then I am here for you.

If you have any questions about ***Easy Fitness for Easy Weight Loss***, here's my personal email address, and feel free to use it: ChrisMorris6217@gmail.com

For more fitness tips and advice, free fitness calculators, as well as developments of this course, please pay a regular visit to https://easyfitnessfor life.net where you can find more Diet Plans, free downloads on the https://easyfitnessfor life.net/free-reports page as well as this free video guide to the exercises:

https://easyfitnessforlife.net/free-exercise-video

www.ingramcontent.com/pod-product-compliance
Lightning Source LLC
Chambersburg PA
CBHW051211250726
48655CB00006B/2356